ABOLISHING THE CONCEPT OF MENTAL ILLNESS

In *Abolishing the Concept of Mental Illness: Rethinking the Nature of Our Woes*, Richard Hallam takes aim at the very concept of mental illness, and explores new ways of thinking about and responding to psychological distress.

Though the concept of mental illness has infiltrated everyday language, academic research, and public policy-making, there is very little evidence that woes are caused by somatic dysfunction. This timely book rebuts arguments put forward to defend the illness myth and traces historical sources of the mind/body debate. The author presents a balanced overview of the past utility and current disadvantages of employing a medical illness metaphor against the backdrop of current UK clinical practice.

Insightful and easy to read, *Abolishing the Concept of Mental Illness* will appeal to all professionals and academics working in clinical psychology, as well as psychotherapists and other mental health practitioners.

Richard Hallam worked as a clinical psychologist, researcher, and lecturer until 2006, mainly in the National Health Service and at University College London and the University of East London. Since then he has worked independently as a writer, researcher, and therapist.

ABOLISHING THE CONCEPT OF MENTAL ILLNESS

Rethinking the Nature of Our Woes

Richard Hallam

Routledge
Taylor & Francis Group
LONDON AND NEW YORK

First published 2018
by Routledge
2 Park Square, Milton Park, Abingdon, Oxon OX14 4RN

and by Routledge
711 Third Avenue, New York, NY 10017

Routledge is an imprint of the Taylor & Francis Group, an informa business

British Library Cataloguing in Publication Data
A catalogue record for this book is available from the British Library

Library of Congress Cataloging in Publication Data
A catalog record for this book has been requested

ISBN: 978-1-138-06764-6 (hbk)
ISBN: 978-1-138-06313-6 (pbk)
ISBN: 978-1-315-16124-2 (ebk)

Typeset in Bembo
by Keystroke, Neville Lodge, Tettenhall, Wolverhampton

CONTENTS

ACKNOWLEDGEMENTS

I am grateful for the astute comments and editorial suggestions of Glenn Shean, Chris Lee, and Gary Brown on early versions of the manuscript, and for innumerable conversations with other colleagues and friends.

1
INTRODUCING THE ISSUES

> Absurd! How can you abolish mental illness? I used to have a mental health problem myself. My great-uncle spent years in an asylum and he was definitely insane!

The title of this book invites the reader to question the meaning of words in common use and to imagine a future in which we stop referring to mental illness. We have given up thinking about people as being 'possessed by the devil'. Perhaps it is time to think differently about how to describe and explain the causes of our woes. At present, we seem content to leave it to experts to declare whether or not we are 'mentally healthy'. The bleak terminology of mental disease or illness is reserved for rather obvious departures from 'mental health', but the idea of pathology is still present in watered-down terms such as 'psychological disorder' or 'mental health issue'. Mental health professionals may rely on little more than answers to a questionnaire measuring 'psychological symptoms' to justify giving out a diagnostic label. If a problem seems to be a 'serious' one, a person's suffering or difficulties will be matched against criteria set out in manuals for diagnosing 'psychiatric illness'.

The idea that the ability to live well has something to do with health and illness has infiltrated our social institutions to a remarkable degree. We have been invited to suppose that 'mental illness' is *illness*, in other words, like a physical illness, something that we either *have* or *don't have*. Mental ill-health encompasses a huge range of undesirable states of being, personal failings, and unacceptable behaviours. I will refer to them using the generic word 'woes', without assuming that the latter share anything in common with respect to their causes or how the woeful person experiences them. Rather than adopt the phrase 'a problem in living', which implies a problem for a particular person, I have chosen the word 'woe' to refer to a state of affairs that is social as well as personal. In its archaic use, a woe was a lament about being afflicted, wretched, or mournful. The thesis of this book is that woes have been medicalised, and recommends that we abandon the concept of mental illness, and imagine a future without it.

This thesis is easily stated but immediately stirs up many questions. In this chapter, I set out the principal issues covered in the rest of the book. It needs to be said straight away that, more than fifty years ago, the psychiatrist Thomas Szasz declared that mental illness is a myth (Szasz, 2010 [1961]). I have therefore devoted a chapter to an analysis of his ideas and the arguments that critics have put forward to rebut them. The opposition Szasz encountered did not simply amount to a spat amongst academics and professionals. The debate about mental illness as a myth goes much deeper than this because a connection between health, illness, and woes has existed in ordinary speech for millennia. Although the concept of mental illness is ancient, it competed with beliefs in divine intervention, witchcraft, and sorcery, which have now largely disappeared in Western societies. The phrase 'mental illness' is now so commonplace that it is assumed to describe a literal state of affairs rather than constituting an explanation. In brief, it attributes a woe to something amiss in the mind or body of a woeful person. In Chapter 3, I explore the historical origins of this myth.

What, then, does it mean to locate the cause of a person's woe in their dysfunctional mind or body? Definitions of disease and illness are controversial, and so this question is not easily answered. However, few people seem to dispute the idea that 'mental illness' is a matter of 'health'. Governments see it as one of their duties to look after the health and welfare of their citizens, and the conceptualisation of woes as illnesses has been accepted across all strands of political opinion. Provisions for 'mental illness' form part of services for physical health and social welfare. I will argue that the concept of mental illness is an example of the medicalisation of woes, and that this has led to mystification about causation, misdirection of efforts, and, on occasions, has usurped human rights. The final chapter of the book critically evaluates the role played by a concept of mental illness in policy documents published recently in the UK.

Mental illness as myth

Thomas Szasz's belief that mental illness is a myth was vigorously contested. He restated his position shortly before he died (Szasz, 2011) and this invoked a scornful commentary (Shorter, 2011), illustrating how little influence Szasz exerted in some quarters of psychiatry. Shorter dismisses the 'weasel word' disorder and places his money on disease. Other experts also express themselves in the uncompromising language of disease. Morgan (2016) states that 'depression is a common and crippling disease', even though he accepts that it 'may be a response to bereavement or other life events'.

Szasz's thesis has been rejected for various reasons. One argument is that mental illness has always been with us, and that we can clearly trace its presence in ancient literature. Another is that no meaningful distinction can be made between diseases of the mind and body, and that the criteria for declaring someone physically ill are essentially the same as ones that define mental illness. Other critics believe that the causes of problematic behaviour must lie in defective genes or diseases of the brain, even though we have not yet discovered them. It is assumed that once we understand the neural basis of mental functions, we will be in a position to define and explain mental illnesses.

None of these objections to Szasz question the concept of mental illness itself. It is as if our woes and suffering must be illnesses because there is nothing else they could be. The idea is so firmly lodged in our way of thinking that to challenge it seems childishly provocative.

Belief in the mythical status of mental illness is quite compatible with an assumption that there is a biological basis to all behaviour and so, in principle, it is possible to reduce all explanations to bodily processes. However, in order to establish solid grounds for describing woes as illness, it needs to be demonstrated that bodily functions deviate (i.e. function differently) when they serve 'normal' and 'distressing or problematic' behaviour. In medical practice, various biomarkers, such as high blood pressure, are used to indicate a state of ill-health of the body. By contrast, there are almost no biomarkers for 'mental illness'. Behaviour that deviates from the norm in a problematic way may be just that – behaviour that is distressing to self or offends others.

It is possible to maintain that mental illness is a myth without denying the existence of a very complex relationship between a person's biological characteristics and their problematic behaviour. In certain cases, it is incontrovertible that problematic behaviour can be attributed to demonstrable bodily dysfunction. Szasz accepted this but drew too sharp a distinction between what he called neurological illness and problems in living. The main reason for arguing that mental illness is a myth is that in the vast majority of these so-called illnesses, the hypothesis of a dysfunction of body or mind lacks supporting evidence. Without this support, there are few grounds for suggesting that the best way to deal with a woe is an intervention directed towards altering the state of the body through medication or other physical interventions. Similarly, when therapy addresses the mind, there is no reason to suppose that this is treatment for an illness or disease of the brain.

There are, of course, differences in bodily functioning between woeful and non-woeful persons, but this is not sufficient to validate a concept of mental illness. Any difference could be an effect of environment or behaviour – that is, what people do, have done, or what they have been, or are, exposed to. They might also indicate a biological predisposition to behave in a certain way. This type of biological diversity is not necessarily a sign of illness or disease. Although a person might be biologically predisposed to exhibit problematic behaviour, a predisposition is not a bodily dysfunction. It is quite likely that the same predisposition could be found in persons who are not in a woeful state. With respect to the category of woes called 'common mental disorders', the evidence that these are expressions of any kind of dysfunction or distinctive biological characteristic is slight or non-existent.

The concept of 'psychopathology' is another expression of the illness myth. It leads us to believe that we should search in the brain or mind for the causes of our woes. It stems from an assumption that 'the mind' is simply a way of describing what the brain does (Hallam, 2012). In fact, there is no widespread agreement on what a 'normal brain' looks like, nor, conversely, a pathological one. It is much easier to describe a pathological liver. So-called neural dysfunctions are often inferred from the social and behavioural effects of an alleged pathology, whatever the brain happens to reveal under empirical examination. It seems that all too often the brain is viewed as a stand-alone organ of the body without regard to its plasticity in changed conditions or its relationship to higher-order processes relating to concepts of person, self, and society. In Chapter 4, I review some biomedical hypotheses used to explain severely depressed mood and consider alternative interpretations of the evidence.

The myth in action

Let us imagine an example of so-called mental illness. A man has made a series of poor career choices, is currently being subjected to bullying by his employer, and all of this has led to a period of low mood, lethargy, spells of crying, and a sense that life no longer has any meaning. Nothing seems to be achieved by calling this episode in his life an illness. The events I have described are not uncommon and the reader might counter with the argument that what I am describing is not an example of a 'real' or 'serious' mental illness. However, whether mild or serious, circumstances like these are often said to result in illness. Everyday conversation abounds with references to 'mental health problems' and 'disorders' (e.g. 'depressive illness', 'eating disorder', 'obsessive-compulsive disorder'). But what has any of this to do with 'health', which we normally understand to be a medical matter? We may suffer 'bouts' of physical illness, but to refer to bouts of depressed mood suggests that something has overwhelmed us for no apparent reason. We 'suffer' from a physical illness because there is often little to be done except retire to bed. A feeling of depression may descend suddenly but it is not imposed like influenza, as a sequence of events that can be given a medical explanation. If our fictional person overcame his depressed mood, would we want to say that he had recovered from an illness? Perhaps he was successful at an employment tribunal, changed his job, moved to a new area, or made new friends. His circumstances changed and he felt optimistic again.

In recommending abolition of the concept of mental illness, I am arguing for a change in the way we describe and explain woes. There are, of course, a multitude of ways in which a person's life can be sent off course and disturb self or others. The reference point for a woe should be well-being rather than health; in other words, a woe hinders the possibility of pursuing a worthwhile life. Woes can, of course, take on a highly idiosyncratic nature, and also reflect unusual beliefs or the influence of destructive relationships. Woes can have complex causes that are not easily put into words. It is not surprising that over the course of human history people have turned to metaphor. Metaphor allows us to express complex intuitions by drawing on common experiences that we understand through direct involvement with the world. Few of us are now farmers but most of our ancestors worked in agriculture. That world has furnished us with a wealth of words and phrases that are still in common use. A person may 'plough their own furrow' in life. Projects 'bear fruit'. Investments are 'harvested'. Illness, in the form that debilitates the body, is something that everyone encounters directly, and when used metaphorically it captures some of the essential features of a woe. If a woe feels like an illness, it is not a bad metaphor. It might convey the sense that the woe is imposed, that it is unfair, and that there is very little one can do about it.

Metaphors should not be taken literally. Financiers do not harvest their investments with a sickle. However, if a woe feels like an illness, it is not surprising that people might look for a credible bodily explanation. When in doubt about the cause of feeling ill, we seek out an expert with relevant training who can identify a cause and offer a remedy. Many woes have effects on the functioning of the body but we do not have to assume an underlying pathological cause. The lethargy of depressed mood need not be attributed to a bodily illness even though it is a bodily experience. The remedies we seek for our woes normally match our suspicion about likely causes. Anyone with a chest pain might wonder whether to consult a cardiologist or an expert in psychological stress.

To assert that mental illness is a myth is to say that illness is a mistaken way of explaining woes. It is as spurious as supposing that a woe has been caused by giving offence to a god or being under the influence of a spell cast by a sorcerer. In practice, in face-to-face dealings between service-users and professionals in the mental health system, the question of diagnosing an illness rarely comes up unless this is required for bureaucratic purposes or it seems necessary to disabuse a person of false information. People usually relate to their woe with the aim of finding a solution to a problem, not to discover their diagnosis. After decades of research into pathological causes of so-called mental illnesses, it must be concluded that this line of investigation has come up with very little. It is time to accept that woes presently called illnesses can have a multitude of causes that lie outside the body. It may not require anyone who is trained in medicine, psychology, or neuroscience to resolve them. In future, we may be able to dispense with the services of a large number of mental health professionals, just as we no longer need experts in casting out spells.

This apparently radical position concurs with the views of people who have been diagnosed as mentally ill. In a recent survey of the attitudes of users or ex-users of the UK mental health service, there was general agreement that a medical model based on deficits and pathology was damaging and unhelpful (Beresford et al., 2016). As the authors state: 'It was clear that language and meaning were very important to people, highly contentious, and that there was no consensus' (ibid.: 24). Participants were not sure that they wanted to be seen as impaired, disabled, or mad. Rather than tackle stigma, users were more inclined to advocate the removal of unhelpful diagnoses. A lack of consensus amongst service-users is entirely unsurprising if mental illness is a myth.

Abolition of the concept of mental illness has to be seen in the context of how society conceives of 'health' and what this means in political terms. Definitions of woes as illness also implicate the medical profession and the legitimate scope of its expertise.

Health as a political concept

There are two distinct everyday meanings given to health in most dictionaries, namely 'freedom from illness or injury' and 'soundness and vigour'. Freedom from illness can be interpreted in two ways. In one sense of illness, a person's health is degraded in a rather obvious way. One feels unwell. In another sense of illness, a medical diagnostic test proves that one is 'ill' or 'not ill' regardless of how one feels. A suspected disorder of bodily dysfunction has been assessed and a verdict given. The second common meaning of health, 'soundness and vigour', is a different sense of feeling well or unwell, and it is compatible with either the presence or absence of a diagnosed dysfunction. A person can feel 'sound and vigorous' without giving any thought to an empirical assessment of their bodily functions. It is simply a state of well-being. Given these nuances of meaning, health, as a political concept, can signify in a variety of ways. For this reason, it seems inadvisable to propose a definition of health that manages to encompass all of these meanings within one concept.

Nevertheless, since 1948, the World Health Organization (WHO) has adopted an all-encompassing definition. It defines health as 'a state of complete physical, mental and social well-being and not merely the absence of disease or infirmity' (WHO, 2017). The clear implication is that disease can degrade health but its absence does not define it. However, by equating health with well-being, the WHO definition opens up the possibility of describing a lack of well-being as a state of ill-health (i.e. illness or disease). In order to be true to distinctions made colloquially, and to clarify what mental illness might mean, it is desirable to put some kind of boundary around a concept of illness/disease.

The WHO definition of *mental health* does not mention either illness or disease:

> Mental health is defined as a state of well-being in which every individual realizes his or her own potential, can cope with the normal stresses of life, can work productively and fruitfully, and is able to make a contribution to her or his community.
>
> *WHO, 2014*

The thesis of this book is consistent with this WHO definition. Mental health, if we wish to use the term at all, is well-being, not the presence or absence of illness or disease. The opposite of being 'well' is a 'woe' or a 'problem in living'. Connell, O'Cathain, and Brazier (2014) call it ill-being.

Very little of what the WHO publishes about mental health is consistent with its own definition. Well-being seems to be tagged on as an afterthought. For example, in its 2011 global survey of mental health (WHO, Mental Health Atlas, 2011), data were collected on the number of people treated and on service-user diagnoses at mental hospitals, general hospitals and outpatient facilities. The amount of money spent on pharmaceutical medications was taken as an indicator of the quality of a country's mental health service. The survey therefore focused on diagnoses of mental illness and their treatment, mainly by members of the medical profession.

Although the WHO Mental Health Action Plan (2013–20) is concerned with human rights and the promotion of well-being, the plan is primarily focused on people who have diagnosed mental disorders. One aim is to 'systematically shift the locus of care away from long-stay mental hospitals towards non-specialized health settings' (WHO, 2013: 16). Another aim is to develop information systems relating to 'a core set of mental health indicators [presumably meaning 'mental *illness*' indicators]' (ibid.: 16). The WHO's chief message seems to be that so-called mental illness causes a loss of well-being, not that mental health (well-being) can be cultivated regardless of so-called mental illness.

It comes as no surprise that the everyday use of mental health terminology mixes up literal and metaphorical meanings. For instance, how are we to interpret the claim made in one recent advertisement for a conference on mental health: 'Sexual abuse in the UK is an epidemic disease which destroys the lives of many young children' (Healthcare Conferences, UK, 2016)? On the one hand, is this hyperbole designed to arouse passions about a serious social phenomenon or, on the other hand, is it really being claimed that both perpetrators and victims are suffering from a disease?

Another example of confusion can be found in the literature of some self-help movements. Rapping (1996: 39) comments that talk of physical or sexual abuse is sometimes conducted in terms of addiction. To construe abuse as mental illness is to take abusers as being addicted to abuse and the victims addicted to being abused. This, of course, conceals the moral, political, and social dimensions of abuse. In reality, perpetrators have committed a criminal offence. It is hard to see how framing abuse within a discourse of health can be justified at all.

In a book on the politics of health, Coggon (2012: 244) argues that health forms part of a philosophy of welfare, not a philosophy of medicine. He views health as a normative concept, not a naturalistic one, and so, for him, health becomes a subcategory of welfare. The risk of defining health in terms of whatever people, normatively, take it to mean is to permit it to mean almost anything at all. It allows people to claim that child abuse is a disease. Coggon is willing to grant that health is 'to an extent subject to scientific understanding' (2012: 246) but this concession does not go far enough. Coggon avoids the contentious status of mental health by failing to mention the topic explicitly except on one page of his entire book.

Although it seems reasonable to disconnect the concept of disease from child sexual abuse, there is no reason to deny the claim (and much evidence to support it) that child sexual abuse can lead to later physical ill-health (Irish, Kobayashi, and Delahanty, 2010). The same psychosocial adversity might cause emotional distress and problematic personal relationships in one person and physical illness in another. Health policy could, as Coggon argues, subsume all legal, social, and treatment provisions relating to child abuse under a superordinate and normative concept of health (or welfare), but it is still necessary to demarcate and justify the roles of the various agencies involved in responding to it. As it is, without a definition of illness/disease that clearly points to the employment of medical expertise, it makes it difficult to open up the field to other kinds of intervention, including ones that are not initiated by the State or undertaken with the aim of promoting 'health'.

Nordenfelt, a philosopher, defines health in terms of a person's ability to realise their vital goals, these being states that are necessary to ensure a person's minimal long-term happiness. He asserts that the attainment of a person's goals can be compromised by 'entities internal to the subject's body or mind' (2007: 57), by which he means impairments, injuries, or defects. He characterises mental impairments as having 'peculiarly *mental causes*, for instance, the mental states of depression and anxiety' (ibid.: 67; original emphasis). This formulation of mental health is vacuous because Nordenfelt simply states the position that mental ill-health has mental causes. It does not help to clarify what mental causes are.

The current investment in biomedicine (intellectual, political, and financial) cannot be attributed solely to a medical definition of health or vested interest in pursuing it. As everyday conversation illustrates, we are all complicit in defining health and illness loosely, allowing all manner of problematic or distressing circumstances to be seen as a health issue. In order to achieve clarity, it would help to distinguish those circumstances for which medical expertise is essential from those circumstances in which medical expertise need play no part at all or merely contribute to the resolution of a woe.

When demarcating the domains of life that rightfully belong to medicine, it is necessary to bear in mind the ambiguous meaning of everyday concepts. The public deserves to know whether a bodily dysfunction can be demonstrably shown to have any relevance when explaining a feeling of illness. We would like to know whether illness potentially means more than just feeling ill or woeful. The public's faith in the medical profession rests partly on the fact that a doctor can demonstrate that our feeling of illness is correlated with bodily signs of dysfunction for which there is a remedy. At present, the remit of the medical profession is much broader than this. For psychiatry, it rests on a belief that the concept of mental illness concerns 'health' and that this makes it a medical matter.

The classification of the causes of woes has profound implications for social policy. We see ourselves as the victims of disease but may blame others or ourselves for woes that are not regarded as diseases. A recent survey of the opinions of medical and lay people in Finland revealed that attributing a person's state of being to a disease was highly correlated with a willingness to devote public funds to it (Tikkinen et al., 2012). Medical personnel were more likely than lay people to view states of being as diseases. Although there was a fair amount of disagreement over many states, there was a consensus amongst lay people that 'schizophrenia' was as much a disease as cancer, and that 'depression' was on a par with malaria. It is apparent that a biomedical understanding of so-called mental illness is widespread.

Definitions of disease and illness

Szasz (2011) defined disease as 'the structural or functional alteration of cells, tissues and organs', but as noted earlier, this definition does not do justice to the complexities of biological and social causation. Szasz's definition resembles one offered by Campbell, Scadding, and Roberts:

> The sum of the abnormal phenomena displayed by a group of living organisms in association with a specified common characteristic or set of characteristics by which they differ from the norm for their species in such a way as to place them at a disadvantage.
>
> *Campbell, Scadding, and Roberts, 1979: 757*

The primary concern of medical practitioners (as distinct from medical researchers) is to have a beneficial influence on the proximal causes of dysfunction in the body, regardless of what has caused the problem in a wider biological, social, or historical sense. For instance, medical practitioners focus on the end result of self-injurious behaviour rather than its causes. When they suspect that the present cause of a problem is 'mental', they refer a person to a mental health professional. They may also advise a person to change their behaviour (e.g. to stop smoking or drinking), but they do not usually consider themselves to be experts in behaviour change. They focus instead on rectifying or ameliorating the proximal effects of smoking and drinking on the body.

A definition of medical practice that focuses on interventions to change the proximal causes of bodily dysfunctions or injuries sums up the bulk of the profession's activities. There are likely to be disputes when specifying criteria for abnormality, such as how well defined and specific the relevant somatic characteristics need to be, and whether the disadvantages they cause are social (e.g. bodily appearance) or biological (e.g. could lead to death).

Lay people tend to define a disease as the identifiable 'cause' of a particular illness. By contrast, for medical researchers, a disease is a theoretical construct that helps them to explain a set of observations. The concept may simply refer to what researchers actually do when they employ the term 'disease' (a nominalist definition). Medical researchers investigate the causal role of past and present biological, environmental, and social events, unlike practitioners who are primarily interested in the consequences of those events on the patient's body. Remote environmental causes, such as the natal and pre-natal environment, are ignored when nothing can be done about them. The way that our genes express themselves in the functioning of our body are influenced by environmental events (Tammen, Friso, and Choi, 2013) and even by the woes of our parents and grandparents. For practitioners, this is chiefly of theoretical rather than practical interest.

For reasons just stated, doctors treat the effects of, say, smoking and drinking, rather than investigate the past causes of these behaviours. Similarly, they treat the dysfunctional effects on the body of past psychosocial adversities. The purpose of abolishing the concept of mental illness is to dispel the idea that woes and distress are caused by proximal events in the body that are analogous to the causes of physical illness. Even though the past (distal) causes of so-called physical and mental illness are often similar, mental illness is a mythical concept when it attributes the present (proximal) causes of a woe to dysfunctional processes in the mind or body without convincing evidence that these processes exist.

The effects of, say, mental fatigue or worrying thoughts, are clearly biological in nature, but it may not be useful to construe their cause as dysfunctions or diseases.

This is not to argue that interventions on the body are unable to relieve the effects of a woe, regardless of its cause, just as many medical treatments relieve pain without addressing the underlying causes of pain. In terms of experience, there is often little to distinguish between physical and so-called mental illness. However, the effectiveness of a medical intervention in relieving distress does not make a woe into a disease.

Psychosocial events, such as the death of a loved one, can have pronounced effects on the body, although the distress (mental and physical) associated with bereavement typically lifts after a period of time. Morgan (2016) believes that bereavement could trigger the 'disease' of depression, a state of affairs that would presumably be signalled by a lack of return to normal mood within a reasonable period of time. The hypothesis he puts forward is that depressed mood could be caused by inflammation (i.e. the body's defences against injury or infection) that goes on to cause damage or disease (as in rheumatoid arthritis). In the case of depressed mood, Morgan believes that inflammation could cause a disease of the brain, which in turn explains the 'symptoms' of depression.

In light of this hypothesis, it becomes clear why the term 'disease' is Morgan's preferred way of describing a depressed mood associated with bereavement. Disease identifies a dysfunctional end-point in the body for which a medical intervention (e.g. an anti-inflammatory drug) could be prescribed. It would be interesting to know if this hypothesis is correct. There is no reason to reject it simply on the grounds that bereavement is a 'normal' process that everyone should be allowed to suffer, any more than the pain associated with childbirth is 'natural' and therefore should not be eligible for relief. However, the inflammation hypothesis is, as yet, unproven. It may eventually suffer the fate of an untold number of other biological hypotheses in psychiatry.

As a medical intervention, an anti-inflammatory drug would focus on a proximal cause in the body. It is not possible, through medical interventions, to change past states of the body. The inflammation hypothesis is therefore uninterested in identifying the causal pathways, initiated by past events, that would have contributed to inflammation in the first place. These are likely to extend far beyond the simple fact of 'bereavement'. Morgan describes depression 'as a disease of the whole person' but apparently he means by this the whole body, not what might have led historically to a person's susceptibility to having an inflamed body. By contrast, psychosocial interventions do often attempt to influence the present impact (mental and bodily) of memories of past events. Where this is possible, there is a clear preference for a psychosocial over a medical intervention because any beneficial effect is likely to be more long-lasting.

Medical practitioners assume that they are dealing with empirical observables, not metaphors. If people diagnosed as depressed do not have an inflammation of the brain, this puts an end to the hypothesis. The present state of medical and psychiatric knowledge is that the vast majority of so-called mental illnesses have not been shown to be the end-point of a known proximal disease process. A disorder is simply stipulated into existence on the basis that it looks like, or is simply assumed to be, the manifestation of a bodily dysfunction.

To recognise that there are remote causes in common between physical illness and so-called mental illness does not mean that we are confused about the end-result. A physical illness usually conforms to a known pattern of disease and has a predictable prognosis if not treated. A cardiovascular disease that has been caused in part by a lifetime of suppressed anger towards a spouse is still cardiovascular disease (Brosschot and Thayer, 1998; Chida and Steptoe, 2009). On the grounds that something like suppressed anger might have the same pathological consequences as, say, a genetic predisposition, Kendell (2004: 41) infers that physical and so-called mental illness must lie on a continuum. A continuum does exist, in principle, in relation to a physical/biological reality, even if we cannot, at present, translate suppressed anger into biological terms. However, a discontinuity exists in so far as suppressed anger does not always lead to cardiovascular disease. The latter is an independently definable dysfunction. So, while acknowledging that there are common causes for many kinds of woe, it is evident that their ultimate consequences can be expressed differently and need different solutions. The way to tackle an addiction to smoking cigarettes differs from the way to treat lung cancer. One is a compulsive habit and the other is a growth in the lungs.

As I intend to use the term, 'medicalisation' can be understood in three senses. In the first, it refers to concepts of health, illness, or disorder in contexts where these terms are misattributions and can only be understood in a metaphorical sense. There is no illness as such and medical expertise is not called for except perhaps to ameliorate (rather than resolve) the distress associated with a woe. Medicalisation in the second sense is simply a preference for dealing with a human woe by means of an intervention on the body. There may be pragmatic grounds for doing so, but psychological or social alternatives are ignored or given low priority. The third sense of medicalisation is individual: a person experiences their woe as an illness when there is little or no reason to offer a medical intervention. This phenomenon is partly related to the other senses of medicalisation, and is reinforced by messages received through the media.

One sociologist who has made a special study of medicalisation declines to offer an opinion on what a 'real' medical problem is. Conrad assumes that we know what 'medical' means when he defines medicalisation as: 'a process by which non-medical problems become defined and treated as medical problems, usually in terms of illness and disorders' (Conrad, 2007: 4). Conrad therefore assumes that medical and non-medical problems can be distinguished but he does not state how this can be done. If 'medical' can mean whatever we wish it to mean, medicalisation is a meaningless concept. Conrad maintains that he is concerned with the 'viability' rather than the 'validity' of medicalisation. The concept of mental illness is certainly *viable* because it is widely adopted in spite of the fact that 'illness', in this context, is a myth. In this book, I will be concerned with the validity of medical explanations in three senses: (1) that a medical intervention is valid when it prevents, corrects, or ameliorates a process or injury that is assumed, with good reason, to be dysfunctional or causes dysfunction; (2) when a medical intervention (although not directed at dysfunction) changes a bodily process, thereby facilitating a person's learning capacity or well-being without too many unwanted secondary effects, and (3) that a medical intervention is only valid when it is offered on a voluntary basis (discounting some rare exceptions to this rule).

Is madness a mental illness?

Madness is not, intrinsically, a medical concept but it describes behaviour that is often incomprehensible or socially unacceptable. When we read of historical examples of madness, we should not infer that 'mental illness has always existed' but only that this projection back in time is a further example of medicalisation. Of course, medical accounts of madness are not new (see Chapter 3).

Although the prototype of mental illness *is* some kind of madness, irrationality, or profound loss of control, this prototype is now applied to all kinds of woes. However, a distinction is usually drawn between 'severe mental illness' and a variety of other common problems that are seen as less serious. Rather than 'mild mental illness', they are usually called 'common mental disorders'. A problem might become apparent when a person checks repeatedly that their front door is locked, when speaking in front of a large group of people invokes great fear, when a person believes they are much too fat when others do not believe this to be the case, when they gamble excessively and lose a large amount of money. Describing these impediments to living well as illnesses or psychiatric disorders does little more than draw attention to the fact a person wishes to act or feel otherwise. They are surface descriptions that do not imply causal understanding. The illness metaphor locates the problem in the individual. It leads a person to assert 'I am (ill, neurotic, addicted, etc.)' rather than 'I am (distressed, affected, not coping, etc.) because of X (worrying thoughts, a compulsion to check, a fear of others, etc.).'

With regard to prototypical madness, the appeal of a medical interpretation is understandable in light of the fact that before the discovery of penicillin, madness was a common sequel to a syphilitic infection. There is no question that bodily disease can have profound effects on mental experience and behaviour. However, the early promise of a biomedical explanation of so-called mental illness has not been fulfilled. With regard to the so-called minor or milder forms of illness, the argument for seeing them as medical conditions is tenuous or non-existent. These 'common mental disorders' are not what first comes to mind when we think about mental illness. However, according to Tversky and Kahneman (1974), a person (or characteristic) that is thought to be typical for a category (that is, a prototype) can bias our thinking about all members of the category. Tversky and Kahneman call this bias the 'representativeness heuristic'. A heuristic of this kind has its uses but it can bias everyday thinking when it ignores how representative the prototype really is. In other words, the bias amounts to ignoring the actual base rates in the population of the person or characteristic concerned. It would be equivalent, say, to having a prototype for a person on welfare as a scrounger and ignore all persons who have a perfectly legitimate reason to make demands on the State.

The significance of 'the mad person' lies in the fact that he or she is firmly established in the cultural psyche, appearing in myths, books, and films (Birch, 2011; Thornicroft, 2006). The image contains only a smattering of reality because the madness prototype is not representative and contains mythical elements. I stress 'madness' because most of what has been written on the subject of mental illness is a discussion of people suffering from 'a severe form' of it. In her book, *Talking back to psychiatry*, Morrison (2005: xi) describes a movement (of consumers/survivors/ex-patients) that is defined by having received a diagnosis of 'serious and persistent mental illness'. In other words, this group does not include 'common mental health problems', which may not be viewed as examples of 'real' illness. In practice, the madness prototype infiltrates all thinking about people diagnosed with so-called minor or mild psychiatric disorders. It is the latter who make up, by a very wide margin, the majority of so-called mentally ill persons. Present diagnostic schemes have left half the population of America potentially diagnosable with a psychiatric disorder at some time in their life (Kessler et al., 2005).

A recent survey of a large random sample of households in the English population found that 44 per cent reported ever having been diagnosed with a mental disorder. For half of this group (around one in five people) the problem was current (HSCIC, 2015). For only 4 per cent of the population did the respondent regard the so-called mental illness as serious. In contrast with the one-in-five figure for a 'current mental disorder', the number of people who were detained involuntarily (usually on grounds that their behaviour is offensive to others or puts them at risk to themselves) is miniscule. In England and Wales in 2014–15, the figure was less than 60,000, in other words, around 0.1 per cent of the population (ibid.). Although most so-called severe mental illness is managed in the community rather than in hospitals, it still represents a minority of all so-called mental health problems.

The size of the group of people who are, or could be, diagnosed with an illness/disorder is also evident from records of prescriptions for antidepressant medication. In England and Wales, the number of annual prescriptions for antidepressant drugs dispensed in the community alone has increased by 28.2 million since 2004 to reach 57.1 million in 2014 (ibid.). This is in a population of around 54 million. Even allowing for repeat prescriptions, the number of people with a diagnosable condition must run into many millions. Antidepressant drugs are prescribed chiefly for depressed mood or for distress caused by 'anxiety', 'panic', or 'obsessions'. On this trend, we may soon reach a point when it is statistically deviant *not* to be taking one of these medications.

Clearly, the number of people who regard themselves as mentally ill does not run into many millions, but the connotation of madness rubs off. A person who has had an official diagnosis may no longer be fully trusted. Unfortunately, early accounts of so-called severe mental illness presented it as a lifelong affliction or permanent identity rather than being episodic and only affecting certain aspects of a person's life. Early descriptions of the diagnosis of schizophrenia in standard text-books were extremely pessimistic: 'Schizophrenia, in its most typical form, consists of a slow deterioration of the entire personality' (Henderson and Gillespie, 1969: 247);

'The disorganisation of personality often results in chronic invalidism and life-long hospitalisation' (Meyer-Gross, Slater, and Roth, 1969: 232). These prognostications were eventually shown to be false (Bellack, 2006) and, in any case, chronic invalidism may have reflected the iatrogenic effects of prejudice, institutional living, and physical treatments. Whitaker (2010) believes that the prescription of psychoactive medications has been a major cause of chronicity. In one study of the long-term outcome of young men diagnosed as schizophrenic, 40 per cent who had stayed off drugs were 'in recovery' 15 years later, and more than 50 per cent were working (Harrow, quoted by Whitaker, 2010: 115). In a group that stayed on anti-psychotic medication, only 5 per cent were 'in recovery'.

It is 'severe mental illness' that mostly shapes political discussion of the need for mental health services. In a book that is 'aimed at all those seeking to develop a national or strategic mental health policy' (i.e. presumably in developing countries), it is argued that mental health 'is of fundamental strategic importance . . . The economic and social burden of mental ill health is massive, and mental illness contributes to poverty' (Jenkins et al., 2002: xiii). The authors claim that it needs to be addressed 'at all levels of society in a range of settings'. They do go on to make a distinction between 'specific forms of mental illness' (i.e. so-called severe mental health problems) and 'minor or moderate psychiatric problems' (ibid.: 2). It is worth noting that in drawing this distinction, the authors switch their terminology from 'illness' to 'problem'. Given the over-inclusive nature of the concept of mental health, the authors' arguments for establishing a mental health service are breathtakingly grandiose.

Prototypical madness remains pivotal in the authors' arguments because they cite a number of international declarations, covenants, and conventions on human rights that are essentially designed to prevent the worst excesses of 'involuntary treatment' of the 'severely mentally ill'. Medical hegemony is asserted in the form of Principle 4 of the United Nations *Principles for the Protection of Persons with Mental Illnesses* that states: 'The determination that a person has a mental illness shall be made in accordance with internationally accepted medical standards' (UN, 1991: 46). Diagnostic manuals of psychiatric disorders at present cover just about every kind of problematic conduct (Gambrill, 2014), and so the scope of any national mental health service is potentially unbounded.

The medicalisation of common woes deflects attention away from their potentially remediable causes and encourages the use of physical interventions in preference to other solutions. Jenkins and colleagues (2002) are certainly not alone in employing a concept of mental health that is loosely defined. Jahoda noted this conceptual mess: 'There is hardly a term in current psychological thought as vague, elusive, and ambiguous as the term 'mental health' (1958: 3). Even though *mental health* is a synonym for well-being, a *mental health problem* is a euphemism for mental illness. As Jenkins and colleagues state, reiterating the WHO definition, 'mental health is more than an absence of mental illness' because it refers to 'a positive sense of well-being and a belief in our own worth and the dignity and worth of others . . . Everyone has mental health needs, whether or not they have a diagnosis of mental illness' (2002: 3). If they are correct, it cannot be denied that a national mental health service would be strategically important – it would cover just about everything that matters. However, it is questionable whether the ability of citizens to live in a 'mentally healthy way' should come within the purview of the State. This question is explored in later chapters.

At present, the concept of mental health has wide-ranging connotations. The UK mental health charity, MIND, states that one in four people are affected by a mental health problem and they give information on more than thirty of them (MIND, 2016). A mental health problem is something you can 'feel' but not 'see', and you might simply know it as 'poor emotional well-being'. In fact, 'How you understand your own mental health, and any problems you experience, will be personal to you.' According to MIND, mental health appears to include any problem that you just happen to have. If so, it is not clear what connection it has to health or to the medical profession.

The inability to say exactly what is meant by mental health plagues both advocates and critics of medicalisation. As already noted, 'mental health problems' are usually subdivided into the 'serious' and 'not so serious' but authors continue to write as if what they have to say applies to both groups combined (i.e. 25 per cent of the population according to surveys). The word 'madness' or its equivalent has been part of the English language for at least a thousand years. Robert Burton in 1621 produced an elaborate four-page synopsis to set out his understanding of the condition he called 'melancholy'. His synopsis was logically arranged into eight general categories, each containing three to six descending subcategories (Burton, 2001: 126). The general causes were divided into supernatural or natural. The natural causes were classified as either primary or secondary, congenital or adventitious, evident (outward) or contingent (inward), necessary or not necessary. Examples of the 'not necessary' causes included bitter jests, scoffs, calumnies, poverty and want, and 'a heap of other accidents, death of friends, loss, etc.'. Burton's 'heap, etc.' encapsulates very well the present-day meaning of a mental health problem.

The merging of the serious and not so serious categories creates an amorphous, mostly stigmatised, section of society called 'the mentally ill'. For instance, Tew (2015) writes about 'mental health and mental distress' but nearly everything he has to say refers to the serious end of this spectrum. In a chapter of an earlier book, he argued that 'mental distress may be conceptualised as both a response to, and an implicit revolt against, experiences of injustice, enforced loss or abuse' (Tew, 2005: 25). This formulation is both too general and too specific. It is too general because mental distress can have much more prosaic causes, and it is too specific because a mentally distressed person is not always a victim in revolt, either explicitly or implicitly. To express this differently, life can be difficult for anyone for a variety of different reasons.

The creation of an amorphous category of the mentally unhealthy is not helped by an imagined link between mental illness and the occasional and fortunately rare occurrence of violent attacks perpetrated by individuals who are deemed insane. This association casts a negative shadow over all kinds of problematic conduct.

For instance, the unprovoked murder of an American tourist in a London square in 2016 by a man who had no obvious motive for doing so, was described in a newspaper as likely to be due to 'mental health issues' (*The Guardian*, 4 August 2016). Fortunately, violent attacks of this nature are extremely rare, especially when compared to violence attributable to alcohol and drug misuse (Harper, 2004).

Living well and 'mental health'

The WHO equates mental health with well-being but in practice focuses on the treatment of mental illness. In Chapter 7, I examine recent literature on well-being and positive psychology and criticise the view that well-being and mental illness are related but independent phenomena. Suffice to say, one valid understanding of living well is the avoidance of unwanted distress or harmful habits, but the latter need not be interpreted as illnesses. Given that most people do not live charmed lives all the time, the concept of mental illness (or mental ill-health) has been recruited to classify together various kinds of failure to achieve a state of personal fulfilment. Instead of following this path, I will be arguing for a piecemeal approach in which each type of woe is considered on its own terms.

A woe is rarely a purely individual problem, even though it is an individual who suffers. A woe could be caused by social arrangements that are expressed in an individual member as a weak point in the system. In this sense, a person's woe can function as a canary in the mine. The circumstances of each human being are unique and therefore their woes tend to be unique. The description of woes as psychiatric disorders largely washes out the individual context and imposes a general pattern. This is also true for physical illness, but with greater justification when a pattern is clearly discernable, identifiable, and explicable.

At some point in life a person is likely to encounter setbacks, problems, or distress. The more the attempt to live well is governed by exacting standards and high ideals, the more probable that difficulties will be encountered. On the other hand, a person who lacks guiding principles is at risk of running into problems through lack of forethought. In other words, living well is not plain sailing and has to be worked on as a continuous project. Old insults and adversities may continue to obscure clarity of vision, paths already taken may have been blind alleys, and to change situations in which problems arise may require difficult decisions, learning new habits, and giving up preferred activities. This scenario does not exclude the disruptive effect of bodily dysfunctions and physical illness. Nor does it exclude the role of conditions that predispose a person to encounter difficulties such as an inherited constitution or temperament, or a physical impairment.

The position I develop in this book is not an attack on psychiatry per se but on its present *raison d'être*. Psychiatry does not have to base itself on a presumption of pathology. Activists opposed to medicalisation have highlighted the harms that psychiatric treatment can cause and the human rights it may violate, but the problem with medicalisation runs much deeper than this and goes beyond psychiatry itself. Nearly everyone is complicit in employing the language of mental illness and in agreeing with legislation that grants psychiatry its power.

This book offers a critique of medicalisation and its potentially damaging consequences. For a person who suffers from or has to endure a woe, a label of mental illness can be confusing. Their woe becomes an 'it', an object that must be passively accepted rather than understood and confronted as something that can be changed. A large section of the population gets to be called 'psychotic', 'depressives', 'obsessives', or whatever the diagnosis happens to be. The point of these remarks is not to magic away human woes but to view them in a different light.

Any attempt to sanitize the concept of mental illness through a well-intentioned effort to encourage people to accept that some of us 'really are ill' only compounds the mystification surrounding the myth. The public is encouraged to be tolerant and to accept that some people are not blessed with mental health. Tolerance is praiseworthy as long as it does not have the unintended effect of entrenching a person in their woe. In any case, tolerance is always selective. It is more easily extended to depressed mood than towards an addiction to Internet pornography. We feel that certain woes are less illness-like than others, but the grounds for doing so are hard to fathom.

If the concept of mental illness were to be abolished, our response to woes would have to be thought through anew. Demystification does not remove the challenges that have to be faced. The issue of personal responsibility looms large. To what extent is it reasonable to expect a person to deal with a woe on their own? Family and friends may provide support, at least in the short term. However, they may be part of the problem. How can other forms of community or peer support be enlisted? At what point does a person admit that they need professional help to solve a problem or even need to seek supervised residential accommodation to ensure their own safety?

In the recent past, pessimism about the future outlook for the 'severely mentally ill' was rife. It was not expected that they would return to full personhood. This pessimism was challenged in the 1960s by anti-psychiatrists and labelling theorists. Their essential message was that 'madness' was a meaningful response to external circumstances and that, if treated as mad, a person would become entrenched in their madness.

One implication of this new non-medical view was that a person was not 'ill' however mad they might seem to others. Their salvation lay in an accepting human response and a changed social environment, which ultimately, it was hoped, would lead to a return to sanity. On these grounds, anti-psychiatrists experimented with small family-type communities in which a person who had lost touch with reality (for shorter or longer periods) was shown tolerance, acceptance, and friendly concern. Madness was seen as a meaningful struggle towards sanity rather than an illness of the brain. This approach to madness demanded that a person be treated first and foremost as a *person* rather than a *patient* in the grip of an illness. On the grounds that an integrated self can only be acquired through social relationships, a mad person had to be treated as fully human.

The ideas of anti-psychiatrists now seem to some critics as hopelessly optimistic. Nevertheless, the question of personal responsibility, and how self-control can be regained, has not gone away. I discuss the general topic of agency in Chapter 5. Free will and personal responsibility were central to the arguments of Thomas Szasz and they resurface in the writings of tough-minded critics of counselling and therapy who are worried about a population going soft and losing its natural resilience. These critics may be wrong in thinking that 'toughening up' is the answer, but any serious advocate of the abolition of the concept of mental illness has to speculate about the limits of personal responsibility and what policies would best help people to confront and overcome their woes. Public policy, without the concept of mental illness, would be left with gaping holes. However, examples of new non-medical initiatives do exist, mostly coming from outside mainstream mental health services (see Chapter 8).

One potential strategy, mirroring that of public health, would focus on prevention. Another would make it easier for private individuals or voluntary associations within the community to take control of their woes as they perceive them. How far a State-funded 'mental health service' would be needed in future is debatable. Many people will continue to rely, as now, on advice and self-help. However, one-on-one advisers (therapists, coaches, change-experts, etc.) need not be funded under the umbrella of health. Given the considerable overlap between physical health and social need/problematic conduct, many of the current statutory services would continue to be needed. The division of responsibility for woes between citizen and State raises many complex strategic issues for policy makers.

To make the task of writing this book more manageable, I will focus on psychiatric diagnoses of depressed mood rather than on all so-called mental illnesses. Critics of medicalisation (and also historians) have tended to make madness their main topic. Madness is somewhat more worrying to the public than is 'depression', although suicide, which is associated with a severely depressed mood, is a leading cause of death. All of the so-called mental illnesses have their own special character and social policy has to take this into account. Efforts to de-medicalise should apply as much to madness as to any other woe. Unacceptable behaviour, especially physical threats to other people, is of particular concern but this is not limited to any one of the current diagnostic groups. The example of 'depression' will suffice for the purpose of critique, and to illustrate how the illness myth blinds us to obvious truths about its relationship to social circumstances. In the final chapter, I describe some new initiatives, and criticise current policy directions.

Summary

A medical vocabulary for describing woes and well-being has, for many centuries, been part of everyday discourse. The causes of woes have been located in a dysfunctional body or mind. There is indeed a complex relationship between a person's biological characteristics and the psychosocial causes of woes, but much of what is known is of theoretical interest only. There is very little evidence for woes as 'medical conditions', and use of the term 'illness' in this respect is metaphorical. The employment of a broad definition of health that joins together dysfunction and well-being has had confusing consequences, with profound implications for social policy. Although bodily dysfunctions and woes share many causes in common, it is desirable to determine what kind of response (expert, lay, or community) would best serve to ameliorate them. The medicalisation of woes has produced a situation in which one quarter of the population is 'mentally ill' and one half will become so at some time in their life. The existence of stereotypes of madness has led to the stigmatisation of a large segment of society. The fiction of 'mental health' should be abandoned and the focus placed on woes and well-being.

References

Birch, M. (2011) *Mediating mental health: Contexts, debates, analysis*. London, Routledge.

Bellack, A. S. (2006) Scientific and consumer models of recovery in schizophrenia: Concordance, contrasts, and implications. *Schizophrenia Bulletin*. 32(3), pp.432–442.

Beresford, P., Perring, R., Nettle, M. & Wallcraft, J. (2016) *From mental illness to a social model of madness and distress*. Published by Shaping Our Lives. Available from: www.shapingourlives.org.uk/wp-content/uploads/2016/05/FROM-MENTAL-ILLNESS-PDF-2.pdf [Accessed 12 December 2016].

Brosschot, J. F. & Thayer, J. F. (1998) Anger inhibition, cardiovascular recovery, and vagal function: A model of the link between hostility and cardiovascular disease. *Annals of Behavioral Medicine*. 20(4), pp.326–332.

Burton, R. (2001) *The anatomy of melancholy*. New York, New York Review of Books.

Campbell, E. J. M., Scadding, J. G. & Roberts, R. S. (1979) The concept of disease. *British Medical Journal*. 2, pp.757–762.

Chida, Y. & Steptoe, A. (2009) The association of anger and hostility with future coronary heart disease: A meta-analytic review of prospective evidence. *Journal of the Medical College of Cardiology*. 53(11), pp.936–946.

Coggon, J. (2012) *What makes health public?: A critical evaluation of moral, legal, and political claims in public health*. Cambridge, Cambridge University Press.

Connell, J., O'Cathain, A. O. & Brazier, J. (2014) Measuring quality of life in mental health: Are we asking the right questions? *Social Science and Medicine*. 120, pp.12–20.

Conrad, P. (2007) *The medicalization of society: On the transformation of human conditions into treatable disorders*. Baltimore, MD, The Johns Hopkins University Press.

Gambrill, E. (2014) The Diagnostic and Statistical Manual of Mental Disorders as a major form of dehumanization in the modern world. *Research on Social Work Practice*. 24(1), pp.13–36.

Hallam, R. S. (2012) Disordered selves. *Contemporary Social Science*. 7(2), pp.197–213.

Harper, D. J. (2004) Constructions of risk in proposals to reform UK mental health legislation. In: Hurwitz, B., Skultans, V. & Greenhalgh, T. (eds.) *Narrative Research in Health and Illness*. London, BMA Books, pp.397–413.

Healthcare Conferences U.K. (2016) Available from: www.healthcareconferencesuk.co.uk/event/1235. [Accessed 14 October 2016].

Henderson, D. K. & Gillespie, R. D. (1969) *Textbook of psychiatry*, 10th edn., revised by Bachelor, I. R. C. London, Oxford University Press.

HSCIC (Health and Social Care Information Centre) (2015) *Prescriptions dispensed in the community in England, 2004–2014*. Health and Social Care Information Centre, 7 July, 2015. Available from: www.hscic.gov.uk. [Accessed 12 December 2016].

Irish, L., Kobayashi, I. & Delahanty, D. L. (2010) Long-term physical health consequences of childhood sexual abuse: A meta-analytic review. *Journal of Pediatric Psychology*. 35(5), pp.450–461.

Jahoda, M. (1958) *Current concepts of positive mental health*. New York, Basic Books.

Jenkins, R., McCulloch, A., Friedli, L. & Parker, C. (eds.) (2002) *Developing a national mental health policy*. Hove, Psychology Press.

Kendell, R. E. (2004) The myth of mental illness. In: Schaler, J. A. (ed.) *Szasz under fire: The psychiatric abolitionist faces his critics*. Peru, IL, Open Court.

Kessler, R. C., Berglund, P., Demier, O., Jin, R., Merikangas, K. R. & Walters, E. E. (2005) Lifetime prevalence and age-of-onset distributions of DSM-IV disorders with national co-morbidity survey replication. *Archives of General Psychiatry*. 62(7), pp.593–602.

Meyer-Gross, W., Slater, E. & Roth, M. (1969) *Clinical psychiatry*, 3rd edn. London, Bailliere, Tyndall and Cassell.

MIND (2016) Available from: https://www.mind.org.uk [Accessed 10 October 2016].

Morgan, P. (2016) We may be able to treat depression with anti-inflammatory drugs. *The Conversation*, 30 August. Available from: https://theconversation.com/we-may-be-able-to-treat-depression-with-anti-inflammatory-drugs-heres-why-64413 [Accessed 10 September 2016].

Morrison, L. J. (2005) *Talking back to psychiatry: The psychiatric consumer/survivor/ex-patient movement*. New York, Routledge.

Nordenfelt, L. (2007) *Rationality and compulsion: Applying action theory to psychiatry*. Oxford, Oxford University Press.

Rapping, E. (1996) *The culture of recovery: Making sense of the self-help movement in women's lives*. Boston, Beacon Press.

Shorter, E. (2011). Still tilting at windmills. *The Psychiatrist*. 35(5), pp.183–184.

Szasz, T. (2011) The myth of mental illness: 50 years later. *The Psychiatrist*. 35, pp.179–182.

Szasz, T. (2010 [1961]) *The myth of mental illness: Foundations of a theory of personal conduct*. New York, Harper Perennial.

Tammen, S. A., Friso, S. & Choi, S-W. (2013) Epigenetics: The link between nature and nurture. *Molecular Aspects of Medicine*. 34, pp.753–764.

Tew, J. (2015) Towards a socially situated model of mental distress. In: Spandler, H., Anderson, J. & Sapey, B. *Madness, distress, and the politics of disablement*. Bristol, Policy, pp.69–82.

Tew, J. (ed.) (2005) *Social perspectives in mental health: Developing social models to understand and work with mental distress*. London, Jessica Kingsley.

The Guardian (2016) Woman killed in Russell Square attack was American citizen (4 August).

Thornicroft, G. (2006) *Shunned: Discrimination against people with mental illness*. Oxford, Oxford University Press.

Tikkinen, K. A. O., Leinonen, J. S., Guyatt, G. H., Ebrahim, S. & Järvinen, T. L. N. (2012) What is a disease? Perspectives of the public, health professionals and legislators. Available from: *BMJ Open*. 2 (e001632), doi:10.1136/bmjopen-2012-001632 [Accessed 10 February 2017].

Tversky, A. & Kahneman, D. (1974) Judgment under uncertainty: Heuristics and biases. *Science*, 185(4157), pp.1124–1131.

UN (1991) *United Nations Principles for the Protection of Persons with Mental Illnesses*. Available from: www.un.org/documents/ga/res/46/a46r119 [Accessed 10 October 2016].

Whitaker, R. (2010) *Anatomy of an epidemic: Magic bullets, psychiatric drugs, and the astonishing rise of mental illness in America*. New York, Crown.

WHO (2017) Constitution of WHO: Principles. Available from: www.who.int/about/mission/en/ [Accessed 10 March 2017].

WHO (2014) Mental health: A state of well-being. Available from: www.who.int/features/factfiles/mental_health/en/ [Accessed 10 March 2017].
WHO (2013) *Mental health action plan*. Available from: www.who.int/mental_health/action_plan_2013/en/ [Accessed 10 August 2016].
WHO (2011) *Mental health atlas*. Available from: http://apps.who.int/iris/bitstream/10665/44697/1/9799241564359_eng.pdf [Accessed 10 August 2016].

2

THOMAS SZASZ AND THE MYTH OF MENTAL ILLNESS

It is important to place Thomas Szasz at the forefront of this book because he was an early and forthright critic of the concept of mental illness. His voice has reverberated down the decades, beginning with the publication of an influential book in 1961 through to when he died by his own hand at the age of 92 in 2012. His major contribution was to describe how, in his preferred terminology, 'problems in living' had been transformed by the profession of psychiatry into a set of diseases or disorders assumed to be dysfunctional states of the body. His further contribution was to supply an alternative vision of how society should respond to people's problems in living, based on his libertarian philosophy. The two sets of arguments are not logically related (Zupan, 1973), and so this chapter is divided into two parts. My aim in the first part is (1) to outline Szasz's position that mental illness is a myth, (2) to critique this position by questioning his grounds for distinguishing mental and physical illness in terms of reasons and causes, (3) to examine several arguments put forward to rebut his thesis that mental illness is a myth, and (4) to make a case for saying that mental illness is a metaphor. In the second part of the chapter, I discuss whether Szasz's libertarian attitude to problems in living is persuasive or credible.

Szasz's book *The myth of mental illness* (1961), influenced generations of psychiatrists, academics, and almost everyone with a professional interest in 'mental health'. It is still in print 55 years later (Szasz, 2010). Although Szasz's numerous writings were an irritant to many in the mental health professions, his continuing influence can be explained in at least four ways. First, despite an early unsuccessful attempt to dislodge him from his academic position, banning him from working in a State hospital, and firing two of his close colleagues, he retained his position as a professor of psychiatry (Leifer, 2016). Although it is fairly easy to discredit criticism from without, it is much harder when the critic comes from within. Second, Szasz developed and expanded his basic arguments through detailed conceptual analysis and historical research. The subtitle of his first book was *Foundations of a theory of personal conduct*. He evidently intended it as more than a blast against psychiatry. Third, Szasz's customary style of writing was penetrating, blistering, but at the same time measured. He provoked a strong response but nearly always one that had to be carefully argued. Fourth, Szasz's challenge to his own profession has not yet been satisfactorily met. He argued that over the last two hundred years, psychiatry has been complicit in medicalising the mind. That the profession in the past has been associated with an abuse of power is self-evidently true. Through his research into its history, Szasz cited authors who condemned themselves in their own words. The illness myth is the foundation stone for attempts to cure underlying 'mental diseases' or relieve their effects. If mental illness is a myth, this rationale is a misplaced basis for any intervention.

A myth is a story we have relegated to history. Its status as a credible account is lost when the beliefs underlying it are replaced by an open-minded attitude or a widely accepted theory. For example, advances in science have destroyed quite a few elements of religious dogma. Most people no longer believe in the myth of Adam and Eve as an explanation for human origins.

Szasz was not initially opposed to psychiatrists offering their services to people who seek them out on a voluntary basis or, as he put it, psychiatric relations between consenting adults. However, he later believed that psychiatry was inseparable from coercion and therefore could not be reformed. If mental illness is a myth, then, according to him, any employment of the concept of mental illness to justify involuntary treatment cannot be supported. Szasz was not opposed to coercion as such; he agreed with punishment for criminal behaviour and had no time for the insanity plea.

Szasz on reasons, causes, and the myth of mental illness

Reasons for acting versus natural causes

Szasz argued that 'the mind' cannot be ill because it is not the kind of thing (an abstraction) that could be said to malfunction. He conceived the mind as comprising our common-sense understanding of a person's reasons or justifications for action. Consequently, for him, belief in the concept of mental illness would involve committing a logical error. A person's acts or mental experiences could be judged as irrational, bad, or compulsive, but only by means of the criteria we use for judging acts as reasonable or morally justified, not with reference to the 'normal functioning' of the human organism. For Szasz, the language of mind and action differs fundamentally from the language of natural causation. He believed that only bodies are subject to pathological processes or injuries causing them to malfunction. His position therefore presupposes that a sharp distinction can be made between mind and body.

The philosophical territory that Szasz had entered has echoes in debates at the beginning of the nineteenth century when reformers wanted to improve conditions in the private madhouses that catered for people who were, at that time, considered to have lost their reason. The English Quakers, William, Henry, and Samuel Tuke, had demonstrated that if a person was treated with respect in a family-like environment, accompanied by prayer and meaningful work, their inner powers of self-control could be restored and they were often able to return to society. This style of managing the mad did not have to appeal to any scientific theory. Its principles could be expressed in ordinary language and they could be justified by successful application.

In any case, no science of behaviour was available at the time to explain madness. Philosophy was still firmly captured by the idea of a separation between mind and body. The concept of a person's mind had developed out of the religious concept of the soul, which was believed to be an immaterial and indivisible substance (Martin and Barresi, 2006). The soul could not be diseased but only 'possessed' by evil forces, a point of view that was, by the early nineteenth century, going out of fashion. The body, by contrast, had for a long time been understood as composed of corruptible material substances. The highly influential philosopher, René Descartes (1596–1650) had not ruled out mind-body interaction, but the direction was conceived as chiefly led from above (i.e. by the mind). The philosophers of Ancient Greece had also raised the soul or mind to a pre-eminent position. Aristotle had defined animate life as a hierarchy of capacities (souls), with only humans possessing a rational soul.

Szasz's arguments resemble those of the Tukes. Through their divinely endowed 'free will', a person could and should take responsibility for the acts they choose in response to their problems in living. They are also similar to the views of an early German professor of psychological medicine, August Heinroth (1773–1843), who viewed psychological disturbances as the result of wrong acts (however generated) that held back a person's soul in its striving for the 'good' (Smith, 1992: 51). Smith points out that later psychiatrists attempted to produce a physiological account of 'mental forces'. This biologising trend in theoretical psychology is not necessarily an example of medicalisation. Szasz was not so much interested in theoretical accounts of brain function, but in the assumption that the brain could be affected by neural pathology, leading to a situation in which the mind is incapable of exercising its natural authority. When this pathology is demonstrable, Szasz would agree that a person is mentally ill in a proper sense of the word. In this kind of illness, the mind is still nominally in charge but there is upward causation from a pathological brain to send the mind off-course.

The possibility of accounting for madness as brain disease was open to physicians in the early nineteenth century in order to advance their claim that they were the natural managers of the mad. In the debate that ensued as to who was best qualified to fulfil the role, the medical profession won out, even though they were, in practice, unable to demonstrate the brain pathology they assumed. As Boyle (2002) explains, the use of moral guidance and gentle persuasion was based on simple principles. However, when in 1845 it became mandatory, under the Lunacy Act, for every county and borough in the UK to build asylums for its pauper lunatics, there was no professional class to fill the managerial roles that were required. Physicians could argue that both a medical and a moral approach were required, and they could supply managers from a long-established and high-status profession.

They also represented the advance of science and the promise of new discoveries. The stage was then set for the medicalisation of woes in the years to follow.

The reason/cause debate can be understood as a carry-over from the distinction between minds (souls) and bodies. At the time Szasz was writing, a number of distinguished philosophers were emphasising the importance of not confusing two types of discourse for explaining human conduct (for instance, Szasz quotes R. S. Peters). Peters makes the point that when we explain why a person does something in particular (such as why they decide to cross the road on a particular occasion), we are implicitly making reference to social norms that regulate conduct: 'Man is a rule-following animal' (1967: 5). He claims that explanations that refer to rules are quite unlike scientific explanations that employ mechanical models. We do, of course, need the mechanics of the body to follow social rules, and sometimes a mechanical problem can explain a failure to adhere to a social norm, e.g. producing illegible writing due to a motor tremor. However, Peters argues that natural processes are never sufficient to provide an explanation for human conduct – that is, to explain 'actions' rather than the mere 'happenings' that the body undergoes. The problem with a natural science explanation of human conduct, as he sees it, is that we could never specify the causal antecedent conditions of an action in an exhaustive way: 'A precise functional relationship could never be established' (ibid.: 18). In his opinion, statements implying norms and standards cannot be deduced from statements about mere movements, which have no such normative implications.

In brief, Peters and Szasz assume that mental life is conducted according to reasons, beliefs, and desires in accordance with social norms whereas bodily (material) life is governed by natural processes. Consequently, a person might have problems in living because they hold false beliefs, want the wrong things, cannot reason sensibly, or cannot exercise their will. Talk of illness would only be justified when a person was physically ill, such as possessing a brain affected by a neurological disease. Szasz adopts the political position that free will is an inviolable component of the status of being human (i.e. personhood). People's bad choices can only be excused if there is unequivocal bodily disease. In practice, he thinks that a lack of 'free will' (bad choices) is often excused by mythical mental illnesses. He opposes the idea that activities of mind can be explained by natural processes on the grounds that this would undermine the idea that we can freely choose to behave in accordance with consciously thought-out reasons and purposes.

Critique of Szasz's exaltation of reason

I will start out from a different philosophical position to Szasz, one that is consistent with the importance we attach to free choice, while not abandoning natural causation as a sensible position to adopt when explaining human behaviour (this argument is elaborated in Chapter 5). I support Szasz's assertion that mental illness is a myth, but for somewhat different reasons.

While Peters may be right that it is impossible to draw moral conclusions from 'mere movements', this does not rule out explaining rule-governed behaviour naturalistically. A great deal can be discovered empirically in order to make predictions about which rule a person happens to follow on a particular occasion. It is true that natural science studies general processes rather than specific reasons for why X did Y. Human conduct depends on all kinds of accidental and contingent events, and explaining their sequences and consequences naturalistically would be an almost impossible task. Nevertheless, it may still be possible in principle and may go much further than Peters imagines. To take the analogy of a unique rock formation, this may be the consequence of past forces of heat and pressure, the minerals present, the effects of water and wind erosion, and the action of living organisms. A skilled geologist is not at a loss to give a well-argued explanation for what she or he sees, even though it represents a unique combination of circumstances and the product of accident. Similarly, what we observe as individual human conduct is not immune to a natural science explanation.

Armed with general principles, we may not be able to predict very precisely the individual rules or shared norms (amongst other causes) that have influenced X to do Y. It would be difficult to generate a complete naturalistic explanation of why Mr Jones crossed the road to buy a newspaper. As Peters points out, two types of explanation need to be distinguished. The rule-based explanation is founded on rules that are shared by the interlocutors. No further answer to the question, 'but why did you want to read a newspaper?', is normally required. This would not be so in a culture in which people could not read. In fact, everyday explanation often appeals to causal relationships of a simple, factual kind. If the interlocutor assumes that Mr Jones is blind, he or she might continue to wonder why Jones is motivated to purchase a newspaper. Naturalistic causal explanations are not weak, and they may have superior predictive power when a person's professed motives are deceptions or self-deceptions.

The strict opposition that Szasz posed between bodily pathology (subject to natural laws) and moral failing (subject only to reason, belief, and will) is not sustainable. Even if we agree with Szasz that mental illness is a myth in the sense that somatic pathology is not discoverable, we are not forced to adopt an explanation of 'problems in living' solely in moral terms. Of course, any 'problem' is an evaluation from a human standpoint, and therefore has a normative dimension. However, this still leaves room for naturalistic explanation, even of moral conduct. We can look to sociology, politics, psychology, anthropology, and of course biology, in a cross-disciplinary perspective that does not require us to adopt the illness metaphor. The fact that a biological level of analysis is always available in principle does not imply that problems in living are the expression of bodily dysfunction. Szasz accepts that brain pathology could have 'mental' consequences, as everyone would agree. What he did not want to countenance is a natural science approach to understanding what for him could only be construed as human conduct – that is, people freely undertaking acts with reason and purpose.

In arguing his case, Szasz seems to employ a valid logical distinction too rigorously. He contrasts a picture of people struggling with moral conflicts with people suffering from disordered bodies, but the causal picture must be far more complex than this.

He appeared to rule out justifiable insights about the causes of woes that can be derived from an understanding of natural processes functioning normally. There is no inconsistency in saying that a causal account could be given for a so-called mental illness while at the same time maintaining that a person's brain was functioning as it was designed to do. The brain could be doing its best when faced with excessive external demands. By changing a person's environment, or how they perceive it, a person's brain may recruit its 'normal processes' to effect a readjustment. In fact, the body's response to a trauma could be interpreted not as signs indicative of pathology associated with disorder (e.g. PTSD) but as a sign of health, just as the body's healing response to a wound is a sign of health.

In so far as woes are caused or maintained by natural processes, it may be possible to develop techniques for changing behaviour that draw upon them. I therefore reject Szasz's assumption that, in the absence of demonstrable brain pathology, woes can only be explained as the outcome of the choices a person has made. He is, of course, right to observe that verbal persuasion differs from changing people's behaviour in other ways. He was also right to emphasise that 'problems in living' are highly individual and relate to unique circumstances, which, often enough, involve existential and moral dilemmas.

The reason/cause distinction in psychiatric thinking

Although it is useful to draw a distinction between different types of reasoning (e.g. based on common sense versus scientific deduction), the distinction between reasons and natural causes can also be misapplied. Marková and Berrios put forward a variant on Szasz's position. On the one hand, they argue that the epistemological basis of psychiatry should lie in language and communication, making it a conceptual undertaking. They suggest that mental disorders are socio-historically constructed labels for various deviations from social norms. On the other hand, and in line with the philosophical assertion that states and processes of the mind are identical to states and processes of the brain, they explain 'mental symptoms' as interpretations and/or articulations of conscious experience or internal states. They go on to write that 'Since all mental states are realized in the brain, then clearly all will have an underlying neurobiological expression, and hence every mental "symptom" will have an associated organic state' (2016: 193). Their position appears to imply that there is a neurophysiological correlate for every deviation from a social norm. This may be true in a trivial sense but they go beyond this by retaining the use of medical terminology, such as 'symptoms'. Marková and Berrios' account of psychiatry as a conceptual undertaking, when combined with mind/body identity theory, therefore does nothing to counter the medicalisation of woes. In fact, it provides a carte-blanche foundation for biomedicine and the pharmaceutical industry.

Other writers refer to different levels of explanation in psychiatry but still retain the concept of mental illness. For instance, Cooper writes: 'It is reasonable to infer that behaviour is probably symptomatic so long as a sub-personal explanation looks like a *better* explanation than does a person-level explanation' (2014: 18; original emphasis).

While it is true that behaviour can look like the product of a sub-personal mechanism (i.e. it is not easily interpretable or explicable in terms of common sense), this is no reason to conclude that the behaviour is a 'symptom' of dysfunction. For instance, behaviour that is irrational or compulsive could be the product of sub-personal processes that are functioning normally. The perception of the behaviour as abnormal rests on social criteria, and the behaviour need not be understood as a 'symptom' of something that is sub-personally 'abnormal'.

There is a temptation to fall back on a concept of illness when a person who shows every sign of taking personal responsibility for overcoming a problem does not manage to do so. Kubie (1974: 500) succumbs to this interpretation:

> Whenever the processes that produce any pattern of behaviour predetermines its automatic repetition irrespective of arguments and exhortations, rewards and punishments, success or failure, even of satiation of instinctual needs, a process has been set in motion that is a process of illness.
>
> *Quoted in Dammann, 1997: 739*

To accept Kubie's account would lead to a reclassification of any recalcitrant behaviour as illness. Heretics burned at the stake could be regarded as having been ill. Kubie also prejudges the effectiveness of psychological interventions such as exhortations, rewards, and punishments. As we now know, but did not know with certainty in 1974, compulsive behaviours (obsessional and compulsive acts) that were once treated by brain surgery are amenable to relearning methods that can be highly effective (Foa, 2010).

Arguments designed to refute Szasz's thesis that mental illness is a myth

The behaviour called mental illness is a universal and timeless phenomenon

The underlying sense of this objection is that mental illness is a 'real' phenomenon. Of course, Szasz and like-minded critics do not deny that whatever is referred to as mental illness represents real problems and real suffering. It is also reasonable to suppose that similar kinds of problematic behaviour have existed in all cultures throughout history. However, a neutral, non-interpretative description for these behaviours cannot be given. Szasz's terminology of 'problems in living' is as much an interpretation as 'mental illness'. This is not the view of those psychiatrists who believe that they are dealing with phenomena that transcend time and culture. According to Pies, naming is irrelevant: 'It is surely misleading to claim that the identification of someone as schizophrenic depends on the social system of institutional psychiatry; names change, but human suffering has changed very little since Avicenna and Burton' (1979: 141).

The proposition that names don't matter is unconvincing. The freedom to name is an exercise in power, and names have consequences. Pies later backtracks and says that 'schizophrenia' is partly invented (ibid.: 142). However, even a part-invention is not an innocent act. Pies raises the example of obesity, which could, presumably, be construed in different ways – as unremarkable, as a sign of a medical condition, or as a form of mental illness. It certainly matters a great deal in terms of social policy (and for the individuals concerned) how it is named. To mark out behaviour by naming it in a certain way changes its social consequences. For instance, while we do not usually mark out masturbation as 'pathological', this was not the case during the Victorian period, with profound implications for the way it was judged morally.

Mental illness and physical illness are identified by similar criteria

The argument here is that mental illness is 'real' illness because the criteria for declaring someone physically or mentally ill are very similar. Peter Sedgwick believes that these criteria are trans-historical and cross-cultural (Sedgwick, 1972, 1982): 'The attribution of illness always proceeds from the computation of a gap between presented behaviour or feeling and some social norm' (1982: 34).

Sedgwick accepts that not all deviations from a social norm are attributable to illness, and that when they are, they relate to a culture's 'theory of the person'. This could not be clearer in the case of Szasz's concept of the person. Sedgwick's argument does not disqualify any society from deciding that mental illness *is* a myth on the basis of its own theory of the person and in accordance with its own preferences for how human woes should be conceived. Hippocratic theories of health and illness, as well as possession by the devil, were constructed in line with cultural assumptions that are now alien to us. In other words, the fact that physical and so-called mental illness share the feature of departure from social norms is irrelevant to the kinds of illness explanation we might wish to make today. Few people argue that physical illness is a myth because we have good grounds for believing otherwise. Sedgwick seems open to various interpretations of the causes of so-called mental illness but cannot dispense with the concept of illness itself. For instance, he cites research by Brown and Harris showing that the origins of 'the psychological illness of depression' are bound up with childhood trauma and the lack of intimate personal relationships (1978: 195). Why then, is it an illness?

Sedgwick's own theory of the person simply presupposes that 'mental illness' is illness. The terms he uses (bearing in mind the era in which he was writing) to describe persons who fall into this category include 'mentally disabled', 'mental deviant' and 'mentally handicapped' (1982: 220–221). At the less severe end of the spectrum, he suggests that 'alternative therapies' might suffice for 'the nearly normal' (ibid.: 223). Most of his attention is directed towards former occupants of mental hospitals, forgetting that the concept of mental illness can medicalise woes for everyone. Sedgwick employs the two terms 'physical illness' and 'mental illness' knowing full well that the reader will understand them differently. He knows that mental illness is a discreditable status because he argues that the mentally ill should be accepted 'in work and social intercourse' (Vice, 1993: 75). He would not have thought it necessary to suggest the same acceptance for the physically ill, although he might have advised against it in the case of contagious illness. You cannot catch a mental illness in the way you can some physical illnesses.

Minds, like bodies, can function abnormally

The concept of mental illness has been defended by suggesting that a normal mind can be distinguished from one that is functioning abnormally. Papineau (1994) compares so-called mental illness to a software bug in an otherwise physiologically intact 'hardware'. If that is so, the term 'illness' is being used metaphorically (as if one's computer is ill when there is a glitch in the software). The brain can only be said to be dysfunctional in a biological sense when the processes mediating a person's woe are intrinsically abnormal (in terms of their innately designed biological function) rather than producing abnormal (socially dysfunctional) outcomes. The existence of biological correlates of our woes is not a sufficient reason to assume that they represent any kind of pathology. Likewise, a computer's hardware is not at fault if its badly designed software does not deliver expected outcomes.

According to Wakefield (1992), it is reasonable to suppose that general processes in the brain or 'mind' that serve thinking, learning, reasoning, remembering, etc., could become dysfunctional in a somatic sense. The relevant processes are conceived as the product of evolved biological systems that ensure normal cognitive functioning, physical survival, and reproduction. If these systems fail to function by reason of neurological disease, Szasz would be in agreement with Wakefield. However, Wakefield's suggestion is that an evolved system could mediate socially dysfunctional behaviour without being somatically dysfunctional. This must be true at times because the evolved systems he refers to presumably contribute to both a good and a bad adjustment to life circumstances (Lilienfeld and Marino, 1995). In the case of a bad adjustment, the evolved biological system might play a decisive role. However, even if the evolved system can cause behaviour that places a person at biological or social risk, this is not a reason to describe this tendency as a disease, illness, or pathology. At best, one could argue that human beings are not designed to function perfectly.

As an example of an evolved behavioural system, we could take the dominance hierarchies that are common in primate groups and are likely to have a strong biological basis. In humans, being too submissive or too dominant may be seen as undesirable. However, whether a person has a problem in this area depends on a close analysis of individual circumstances and local social norms. For instance, highly aggressive, risk-taking acts might be appreciated when directed against the enemies of a community under threat. Assertiveness training has become popular as a set of techniques designed to encourage or restrain individuals at either end of the dominance continuum. These problems are not illnesses in the sense of a dysfunctional brain system, and the significance they have acquired in democratic societies is a reflection of new human rights.

As Boyle (2002: 226) argues, it is not enough to point to a function like memory and to declare that when memory is dysfunctional that this demonstrates the existence of mental disorder. There are many circumstances in which memory is defective, but we would not want to attribute them all to illness or somatic disorder. In some cases, such as memory loss associated with ageing, this seems justified. It is not unreasonable to suggest that there are cogent medical approaches to some forms of memory defect. For instance, researchers have proposed using stem cells to restore neural functioning in the brain's memory centres (Choi et al., 2014).

However, to be confident that a concept of pathology fits the circumstances, it is necessary to theorise about the mechanisms underlying memory and to show how they are malfunctioning. It would also be necessary to argue that they led to a condition that people wanted to redress. There are many examples of somatic dysfunction that a person, or society in general, decides to ignore. Moreover, it is not easy to single out pathology from other types of explanation, e.g. distinguishing between the case of someone whose memory is dysfunctional on account of ageing or alcohol poisoning and the person who cannot remember what happened at the time of a trauma or forgets personal events that might show them up in a bad light. In order to justify a medical intervention, it is desirable to have a theoretical basis for changing a memory process. It is not sufficient to propose an abnormal neural or mental process unless the underlying abnormality can be identified independently of the distress that someone happens to report. The term 'disorder' seems appropriate when there are clear empirical somatic referents that have the nature of a dysfunction. However, even when these are demonstrable, they would not constitute an illness unless they caused distress or problems.

Demonstrable abnormalities of cerebral function do not always have socially problematic consequences. A person with manifest memory loss commonly 'confabulates', that is, unwittingly covers up gaps in memory with plausible reasons for their apparent forgetfulness. A particularly striking example of the interaction between a neural deficit and how it impinges on social reality is what is called 'visual hemineglect' (Cooney and Gazzaniga, 2003). In this condition, a person fails to perceive one half of their visual field and they may also neglect any memories of how this half-field used to function. Consequently, when looking around, a scene appears normal, and rotating the head simply brings objects into view. In some other rare cases of neglect, the denial of a problem seems quite bizarre, such as when one side of the body is paralysed. When asked to explain why they are incapable of performing a task requiring two hands, a person might simply claim 'I did not want to do it.' They do not appear to be aware of their manifest disability and therefore do not regard themselves as in need of treatment, even though there are good grounds for assuming a neurological disorder. Of course, the disorder may be morally problematic for others if it leads to, say, unsafe use of machinery or a vehicle.

These are rare conditions but they illustrate a general point. A person could be adamant that their explanation for acting was genuinely rational and purposeful when, assuming that methods were available for analysing how the brain normally functions, it could be shown that there were deviations from optimal neural functioning. Even with clear criteria and evidence for pathology, we cannot say that a person is 'mentally ill' in the sense that they are suffering from a disorder of something. It is probably rare, in fact, for anyone to be on 'top form' neurologically speaking. In one striking example, a white-collar worker, to all appearances a successful ordinary member of society, was discovered at autopsy to have a highly anatomically abnormal brain (Feuillet, Dufour, and Pelletier, 2007).

The competence of a person's behaviour is judged against social criteria that permit a certain degree of latitude. If there are, in reality, biological malfunctions in one area or another, these may be compensated by other systems. In certain cases, a failure to meet social expectations can be attributed to a poorly functioning mental process (e.g. a learning difficulty). However, a person diagnosed in this way might still deny that they were 'ill' or 'disabled'. The risk associated with defining so-called mental illnesses as 'anomalies' of mental or neural processes is that the definition of a woeful state is taken out of the hands of the person who is supposedly suffering. The research strategy of looking for possible brain disorders that underlie so-called mental illnesses therefore raises ethical issues. To take one organ, the brain, as the sole key to understanding all of the multiple levels of human existence, is philosophically and scientifically flawed (Greenberg, 2011; Paris and Kirmayer, 2016).

Kendler, a psychiatrist, believes that each mental illness could correspond to a 'mind-brain homeostatic property cluster', an interconnected network within mind or brain systems. He understands a disorder as an 'emergent syndrome': 'What makes each psychiatric disorder unique are sets of causal interactions amongst a web of symptoms, signs and underlying pathophysiology across mind and brain systems' (2016: 9).

Kendler admits to an 'underlying commitment to the reality of psychiatric illness' (ibid.: 12). Given that the brain mediates all behaviour, there are bound to be brain states that correspond with each so-called psychiatric illness. However, it is unclear how the networks Kendler refers to could be researched without a prior belief that the 'property clusters' he proposes correspond to psychiatric disorders. It might be concluded from research into them that this way of classifying the clusters was entirely inappropriate, especially if the networks excluded events and processes beyond the boundary of mind and brain.

The US National Institute of Mental Health has recently produced new guidelines (Research Domain Criteria – RDoC) to give direction to future grant proposals (Insell, 2013). These guidelines do not focus on somatic dysfunction as such because they broaden out the search for underlying causes to include psychological processes that lie on a continuum with normal functioning. It proposes a number of domains and levels of analysis that are best described as psychobiological, because they refer to systems relating to constructs such as threat, reward, loss, attention, memory, arousal, attachment, and theory-of-mind. These constructs can be investigated at different levels, from the most reductionist (e.g. molecular, genetic) to the most general (e.g. social and experiential). However, as Paris and Kirmeyer note in relation to the higher levels:

> Yet, the RDoC system is presented in a way that gives little detail about these levels and therefore does not seem to encourage researchers to study

> mind, behavior, or experience unless they are also able to measure some correlative neural activity.
>
> *Paris and Kirmeyer, 2016: 29*

The new research strategy may produce findings that contribute to the explanation of woes but the strategy, as a whole, only makes sense when it retains a concept of psychopathology. By removing an emphasis on suffering, the strategy fosters a general search for anything that might predispose a person to suffer. Virtually everything connected with human existence becomes relevant to understanding 'psychopathology'. In practice, the search seems to be narrowed to mind and brain, with little sign that this new approach will focus on the social, cultural, ethical, or political context of woes.

Mental illness as metaphor

Szasz's definition of illness as 'the structural or functional alteration of cells, tissues and organs' (Szasz, 2011) has been rightly criticised as too narrow and too reliant on a separation between mental and bodily processes. Moreover, his employment of the reason/cause distinction does not provide a good foundation for his argument that mental illness is a myth. Notwithstanding these criticisms, it can still be argued that mental illness is a myth because there is something that we reliably call 'real physical illness'. Mental illness as a metaphor derives its force by borrowing from literal illness. For this metaphor to have been so widely adopted since antiquity, there has to be a literal meaning of illness, equivalent to literal butterflies when we refer to butterflies in the stomach. A prototypical physical illness, as we understand it and experience it, is more or less as Szasz defines it, and consists of disabling or distressing effects that are (or could reasonably) be attributed to some underlying pathology, lesion, or dysfunction that affects a bodily process. The distinction between physical and mental illness seemed obvious to Robert Burton writing in 1621 (Burton 2001 [1621]), presumably because he could detect differences in their phenomenal description or causes.

As I argued in the introductory chapter, the distinction we make between physical and so-called mental illness revolves around *proximal* causes in the body. There is likely to be a broad overlap in the *distal* causes that lead to physical illness and the states of affairs I have called woes. Common antecedent causes can have quite dissimilar consequences, all of which may also share the feature of suffering and negative evaluation. A key difference is the type of professional help thought to be appropriate for dealing with the proximal causes of suffering. In the past, the physician's remit was far wider than it is today and was justified by theories that embraced cosmology, spirituality, and holistic health. This is no longer the case for Western medicine. Medical practitioners are now primarily concerned with the proximal causes of bodily dysfunctions. The sub-discipline of psychiatry has the same historical roots but is only loosely integrated with the profession of medicine as a whole.

As Boyle (2002, Chapter 4) points out, we normally accept that a physical illness has been correctly identified when it is founded on a valid scientific explanation of its proximal causes. In other words, the disease or disorder that is assumed to be causing the symptoms allows predictions to be made about what other signs can be medically observed, what laboratory tests will show up as positive or negative, and what treatments are likely to be curative. Medical knowledge advances on the basis of evidence, and the modification of non-somatic factors that have a bearing on disease (behaviour, environment, etc.) is usually left to others.

It remains open to medical practitioners to produce a definition of illness that includes suffering, behavioural deviation, in addition to dysfunction of somatic processes. Pols, a psychiatrist, names this the biopsychosocial definition of illness. He criticises the biomedical concept for focusing solely on bodily dysfunction. In his opinion, whether or not there are 'physical aberrations in schizophrenia' is 'an ardent and rather fruitless controversy' (2005: 136). He points out that many physical anomalies are not signs of present or past disease. He says that they only count in classification when they are 'demonstrable, relevant and have the nature of a process'. He declares that biomedical criteria, in themselves, are not sufficient to define illness.

If Pols's biopsychosocial definition of illness is adopted, virtually any form of social deviation could be called an illness. He admits:

> Psychiatry scarcely utilizes the techniques and methods of somatic specialities, respective of medical examination as well as treatment. The boundaries are indistinct and determined more by daily practice, experience, and sometimes local conditions, in short, by pragmatic arguments rather than principles.
>
> *Pols, 2005: 137*

The case for abolishing the concept of mental illness is precisely that the practices it engenders are indeed unprincipled and, in pragmatic terms, no longer convincing.

One objection to the distinction I have drawn between real illness and metaphorical illness is that they share several features in common. When arguing about similarities and differences, it is always possible to focus on one rather than the other, with the result that the debate has no factual resolution (Pickering, 2006). However, psychiatric researchers are unrelenting in their search for biomarkers of 'mental illness'. If they were happy to come up with a broad, all-encompassing, definition of illness (physical or mental), that took account of the fact that cultural values and deviation from a normative ideal enter into any judgement of illness, all the fuss generated by Szasz's ideas would soon be forgotten. Instead, he was met by angry rebukes because the connection between psychiatry and medicine is fundamental.

Pickering (2006: 78) also points out that scientists may choose a metaphor because it illuminates a phenomenon, and he gives the example of the body as a machine. He argues that calling madness an illness could be seen as a creative leap of the imagination. Perhaps this was so at some time in our history but the metaphor is no longer scientifically useful, even though it is widely employed. It now influences the way that most people habitually think, and the concept can be rejected for sound reasons. Szasz's views generated considerable heat because there was much more at stake than the choice of a useful metaphor for scientific speculation.

Malingering and somatisation

If we accept that some illnesses are 'genuine' physical illnesses, then a malingerer is someone who pretends to be ill for some personal advantage. Szasz extended this idea to people who pretend to be 'mentally ill' for similar motives. A person who 'somatises', by contrast, genuinely believes that they are ill, and there is no reason to doubt that they are genuinely suffering. However, the medical expert is unable to detect a somatic cause and usually believes that the suffering, which is expressed somatically, has its origins in psychological or social circumstances rather than pathology.

For more than a century, sociologists have taken an interest in the way patients and their doctors respond to illness, and Szasz accepts the validity of the long-standing distinction that has been made between illness and disease. Illness has been theorised as a social status in which a person (and those surrounding him or her) acknowledges that a deviation from ideal health is sufficiently marked for them to be excused their normal obligations. They are encouraged to seek medical advice and, having done so, are expected to behave accordingly and accept medical treatment. People do not always take their illnesses sufficiently seriously and some public health campaigns target a lack of awareness of the hazards of ignoring their causes. We have, then, four categories of health. The lucky individuals are those without signs of pathology or dysfunction who have no concern that they are ill. Second, there are those who are diagnosed as ill, accept the fact, and take appropriate action. Third, there are those who deny they are ill (despite evidence of dysfunction) or they simply decide to ignore evidence that this is the case. Finally, there are those without any signs of pathology or dysfunction yet still feel themselves to be ill. As noted above, they may be malingering. Alternatively, they may believe that they have an illness because they have convinced themselves that they are ill or they simply feel ill. They may believe this because it is what they have been told or believe it despite what they have been told.

In a thorough review of sociological theories of health and illness behaviour, Young (2004) incidentally reveals, through not mentioning the topic, that sociologists of health have not given much consideration to the existence of mythical illness. In the theories that Young reviews, sociologists are chiefly concerned with a 'response to symptoms' or 'the perception of illness'. There is a clear implication that illness is something you have rather than invent. Young presumably fails to consider mythical illness because it *is* a fiction according to the tenets of Western medicine. A mental illness is a construction placed on a state of affairs that could have been perceived otherwise.

On Szasz's account of disease, people who are called mentally ill are either malingerers, deceived, or self-deceived. Of course, illness is not a bad metaphor. A person may have very good reasons for suffering mentally or feeling ill in their body. They may lack energy, mope around, be unable to sleep, pace up and down, or lack an appetite for food. So-called mental illness does involve suffering. Szasz distinguished between mental and physical illness on the grounds of a correct explanatory model (together with honest reporting), not on how illness is experienced by the person concerned. He defines some woes as 'physical' on the basis of their cause (e.g. a blow to the body or disease pathology) and others as 'mental' because they communicate a message through symptom-like signs. Szasz must be right that much of what we call mental illness can be interpreted as an attempt at meaningful communication. The criticisms I made earlier of Szasz do not undermine his argument that the concept of mental illness involves a metaphorical use of language.

Abolition of the concept of mental illness: Szasz's libertarian alternative

Abolition of the concept of mental illness would still leave us with the question of what to do about woes or problems in living (apart, that is, from not treating them as illnesses). The impression Szasz gives is that a person solves a problem as it arises and takes the consequences if the attempt fails. He would have everyone face up to their own problems because, for him, individual responsibility and 'free will' are sacred.

With regard to the tragic nature of existence, Szasz acknowledges that a person has to create meaning in a life that routinely contains suffering. How we come to terms with the tragic element is, for Szasz, answered by his own political beliefs. These are a more extreme version of a principle that most people accept, namely, that everyone is, by default, 'free to choose' and is therefore responsible for their own acts. However, acting responsibly is clearly much more difficult for some people than it is for others. A country with a welfare system recognises this and attempts to create a level playing field. People are assisted when they have difficulty in meeting expectations and, in the case of a complete failure to take responsibility (or when a person constitutes a serious danger to themselves or others), coercive methods are employed. In the grey area between a capacity and an incapacity to assume personal responsibility, there is a variety of different options for achieving the goals of personal welfare, fairness, and social cohesion.

One problem with Szasz's categorical style of thinking is the practical difficulty of distinguishing between the person whose brain disease renders them unable to make moral choices and the morally irresponsible person who disguises their immoral acts by claiming to be ill. There are also members of society who, because of their experiences or impairments, are seen as being liable to act against the law, and therefore should be treated more leniently. Szasz seems to resolve these moral dilemmas by stating that every person qualifies as a moral agent, regardless of whether we want to assign praise or blame:

> Holding a person responsible for his act is not the same as blaming or praising him for it: it means only that we regard him as a moral agent . . . Conversely, holding a person not responsible for his act by reason of mental illness means that we do not regard him as a (full-fledged) actor or moral agent.
>
> *Szasz, 2007: 15*

Szasz regards all so-called mentally ill persons as moral agents, and assuming that there is no evidence of neurological disease, he would have them face up to the consequences of all their acts. Mental illness is not a legitimate excuse for wrongdoing. Szasz argues that a person who claims that 'God's voice commanded me to murder' is not to have no reason for murder, it is to want to kill but to disavow the intention. The person is a 'victimizer rationalizing his action by attributing it to an irresistible authority' (ibid.: 16).

Given the possibility of undiagnosed somatic pathology (and the assumption that psychiatric disorders are real illnesses), it is not surprising that expert witnesses called in to give evidence at criminal trials often argue for leniency (or involuntary hospitalisation) in cases of supposedly 'uncontrollable impulses' to murder.

If we accept Szasz's opinion that regarding a person as a moral agent does not necessarily lead to praise or blame, it may still be a good policy to punish him or her even if we do not know what has caused the person to offend. The policy may deter others (even though some persons found guilty should really have been judged as 'ill'), or it may help others to reform. As a general policy, some errors of judgement will be inevitable. Szasz expounds a version of the Western cultural concept of the person, which, for him, logically entails certain consequences. He sums up his position as follows: 'The point is that attributing or refusing to attribute moral agency to the Other is a matter of both fact and tactic—a decision that depends not only on the Other's abilities but also on our attitude towards the Other' (Szasz, 2007: 18).

According to this rather ambiguously phrased statement, we might be lenient with an offender on the basis of, say, their level of intelligence, gullibility, or irregular abusive childhood, or be tough because we wish to set an example. Szasz leans towards an interpretation of so-called mental illness as malingering because he sees it as a dishonest evasion of personal responsibility for problems in living. He construes a complaint of mental illness as a purposive act, although he seems to admit that a person captured by the language and mythology of mental illness might succumb to it involuntarily. As an act that is motivated by a goal, Szasz assumes that feigning illness yields some kind of personal advantage: to receive sympathy, to be let off onerous obligations, to qualify for a pension, or, in its more subtle forms, to engage in the sick role with the explicit sanction of a mental health professional. Szasz points out that the professional also gains from the myth. It justifies a lucrative occupation (as it must have done for him) and, in those cases that fall under mental health legislation, it grants the power to impose a diagnosis and treat a person against their will.

If the concept of mental illness were to be abolished, Szasz must be correct in assuming that some people would exhibit problems in living that would need to be sanctioned by the criminal or civil law. However, the basis for doing so could be justified pragmatically according to their actual consequences, rather than being seen as treatment for mental illness.

With regard to psychotherapy for ordinary problems in living, Szasz regarded the myth of mental illness as serving the interests of both the patient and their mental health professional. For the patient, he considered it to be a way of evading responsibility for dealing with the real causes of problems. For the professional, the benefit accrues by fulfilment of a paid role sanctioned by law and widespread acceptance of the illness myth.

Resistance to medicalisation has largely been founded on people's experience of involuntary hospitalisation and the power, enshrined in mental health legislation, to determine how woes are defined. Involuntary treatment was a major concern to Szasz and it motivated a large part of his written output. However, the vast majority of people diagnosed as mentally ill acquiesce to treatment on a voluntary basis. I include here the person who attends their general physician and receives a prescription for a psychoactive drug. The question of whether the person should be rigorously examined for a somatic disorder rarely comes up, although tests may be conducted to exclude causes such as a malfunctioning thyroid gland or a food allergy.

Szasz's political position raises at least two questions about the patient's perspective: whether he or she knowingly or unknowingly is evading responsibility, and whether, if the causes of a problem in living were to be revealed, they could reasonably be expected to take responsibility for resolving them. Szasz had definite views on how psychotherapy should be conducted, and I think that few people would accept his uncompromising position on personal responsibility. As regards the professional, we can ask whether she or he really believes in the myth of mental illness (and consequently always offers a medical treatment), or whether they see their role as helping a person to uncover the reasons for their problems in living and provide assistance in resolving them. Present mental health services combine both of these approaches.

Szasz expands on the implications of his adoption of the reason/cause distinction in a chapter entitled 'Persuading persons: Rhetoric as remedy' in *The myth of psychotherapy*. He asserts that the language of science and technology is only seemingly value free, and he goes on to view technology as potentially 'a threat to human freedom and dignity' (1988 [1978]: 19–20). He maintains that one advantage of rhetoric, unlike arguments that use the abstract and universal concepts of science, is that it 'is always concerned with the particular and the individual' (ibid.: 19). Although Szasz is right to point out that rhetoric is often dressed up as science, it is pessimistic to suppose that it is impossible to distinguish rhetoric from scientific claims. Szasz saw psychotherapy as often being a form of 'base rhetoric' that uses false reasoning, concerned with power, rather than being an example of 'noble rhetoric', that seeks to persuade through showing us a better version of ourselves. Szasz seems to regard any application of science in attempts to overcome woes as an example of base rhetoric. However, it is unrealistic to disbar science from attempts to understand human conduct or to change it. A person who is trying to comprehend their woe might want to use scientific reasoning and factual evidence to get a clearer picture of what might have led them into difficulty. In some cases, the answer might indeed be found in a bodily disorder they had not suspected. Moreover, evidence exists that can guide a person about the consequences of making a change to their behaviour, including, for instance, the pros and cons of taking a psychoactive drug. In any case, noble rhetoric has to appeal to what we factually believe to be the case, drawing upon universal, abstract concepts. The particulars of our life cannot be understood only in terms of other particulars. In fact, particulars are often pinned down by identifying them as a unique intersection of abstractions.

Because Szasz believes that psychotherapy is 'rhetorical talk', he seems to rule out natural causal influences of the relationship (beneficial or detrimental) of a therapist upon their client. Nor, presumably, would he regard as legitimate any intervention based on a natural science rationale, in other words, any technique that operates 'naturally' with mental consequences. According to him, this would violate a person's freedom of choice unless, presumably, that person had freely chosen to have their mind altered in this way. For Szasz, to allow that the 'mind' can be changed by techniques based on natural science undermines his strict separation between reasons and causes. Szasz's insistence on free will presupposes that we can distinguish between 'free' and 'determined' causes of action. While there are solid grounds for defending people's human rights and freedoms, it is unclear what any of this has to do with a natural science explanation of free and determined behaviour (see Chapter 5).

Szasz's alternative to the employment of a concept of mental illness is to strengthen and enforce the civil right of each person to choose how to live their life and take responsibility for the consequences of their own choices. As he phrased it in 2010, 'freedom is more important than health' (Moncrieff, 2014). He was opposed to communitarian or statist responses to woes. He emphasised the rights of a citizen in a democracy, through their 'free will', to resolve their 'problems in living' in whatever way they choose. He champions a right to refuse 'medical labelling' or 'coercive treatments'. Of course, if a person chooses to ignore the effects of their own behaviour on others, he or she might have to bear the full brunt of the civil or criminal law. Moncrieff argues that decisions about a person's capacity to make rational decisions are always going to be subjective but suggests that removing the link with illness 'might make the nature and purpose of coercive interventions in psychiatry more apparent' (2014: 5). She suggests that the community as a whole should take responsibility for things done to control people designated mentally ill, and also sample the opinions of the diagnosed mentally ill when making these deliberations. How this could be achieved, if feasible at all, is yet to be worked out.

Szasz (2003) takes the ethics of his own psychiatric practice to a place where I think few would be willing to follow. He removes himself from any idea of doing or giving something to a client, and describes what he does as 'existential intimacy', comparing it with marriage or friendship. At the same time, Szasz sees therapy as a straightforward financial transaction in which listening and talking is exchanged for a fee on an entirely voluntary basis. The client contracts to be entirely responsible for whatever they choose to do, even if this means taking their own life. The therapist has no obligation to consider the protection of third parties or the community. In fact, he thinks the therapist should 'abstain from meddling into the client's affairs and life' (ibid.: 53). At this point Szasz's position sounds faintly ridiculous because he was, himself, clearly prone to be very judgemental of others. In the same article, he condemns R. D. Laing for having allowed his 24-year-old daughter, distraught over the ending of a love affair, to be committed to a mental hospital and then be treated with electro-convulsive therapy (ECT). He similarly accuses Jacques Lacan of prescribing shock therapy for Dora Maar, the lover whom Picasso rejected and entrusted into his care. His forthright expression of a moral position was likely to have been a habit that was conveyed to his clients, however much he just 'talked and listened'. I assume that if Laing or Lacan had been his patient, he would have found it very hard not to meddle just a little. 'Meddling' has a negative connotation, and challenging or debating would more accurately describe what therapists do. The listening and talking that goes on in therapy is not simply an entertaining form of after-dinner chat. Clients do seek out therapy in order to be meddled with, in relation to the problems they present.

Szasz's views on personal responsibility and his endorsement of the justice system to curb deviant or troublesome behaviour is ultimately a statist solution to running a society that is tolerable for the majority of its members, given that it is one way of dealing with disruptive persons. However, the legal system can be as biased in favour of the powerful as can psychiatry. For instance, a legal challenge is often unavailable due to its cost. I suggest that there are as many constructions of, and solutions to, the woes presently attributed to mental illness as there are types of problem they entail. Szasz's arguments about mental illness as a myth can be accepted without taking up his own forthright alternative to it.

Szasz is most convincing when he argues that the State co-opts the myth of mental illness when devising, through legislation, systems of social control. For this type of social control, he adopts the phrase 'the therapeutic State' (Szasz, 1984; Leifer, 1990). The concept of mental illness then becomes an officially sanctioned form of mystification. For example, people who are unemployed or otherwise socially disadvantaged may be encouraged to believe that they are suffering from a mental disorder that prevents them from successfully obtaining work. Their welfare benefits may be made conditional on entering training programmes designed to help them 'shape up' psychologically (Friedli and Stearn, 2015).

Summary

The views of Thomas Szasz on mental illness as myth are examined and critiqued. His strict distinction between a person's reasons and motives for acting, and the natural causes of behaviour, cannot be sustained. However, various arguments put forward to refute the thesis that mental illness is a myth do not succeed. Despite similarities in the way concepts of physical and mental illness are used, the central feature of significant somatic dysfunction distinguishes them. So-called mental illness can feel like illness and be expressed somatically, and this may explain why the metaphor of illness has become so entrenched. A key policy issue is how the causes of mythical illness are best addressed. Szasz's approach to the problem is over-reliant on concepts of free will and personal responsibility. It is argued that natural science can play a part in understanding the causes of woes and can sometimes provide technical resources for their resolution. At the same time, Szasz's belief that woes are primarily individual and involve failures of practical and moral reasoning is justified. Psychotherapy is primarily a form of rhetoric, although it can also make use of the knowledge and techniques of natural science.

References

Boyle, M. (2002) *Schizophrenia: A scientific delusion?* 2nd edn. Hove, E. Sussex, Routledge.

Brown, G. W. & Harris, T. O (1978) *Social origins of depression: A study of psychiatric disorder in women*. London, Tavistock Publications.

Burton, R. (2001 [1621]) *The anatomy of melancholy*. New York, New York Review of Books.

Choi, S. S., Lee, S., Kim, S. U. & Lee H. J. (2014) Alzheimer's disease and stem cell therapy. *Experimental Neurobiology*. 23, pp.45–52.

Cooney, J. W. & Gazzaniga, M. S. N. (2003) Neurological disorders and the structure of human consciousness. *Trends in Cognitive Science*. 7, pp.161–165.

Cooper, R. (2014) *Psychiatry and philosophy of science*. Abingdon, Routledge.

Damman, E. (1997) The myth of mental illness: Continuing controversies and their implications for the mental health professions. *Clinical Psychology Review*. 17, pp.733–756.

Feuillet, L., Dufour, H., & Pelletier, J. (2007) Brain of a white-collar worker. *The Lancet*. 370(9583), p.262.

Foa, E. B. (2010) Cognitive behavioral therapy of obsessive-compulsive disorder. *Dialogues in Clinical Neuroscience*. 12, pp.199–207.

Friedli, L. & Stearn, R. (2015) Positive affect as coercive strategy: Conditionality, activation and the role of psychology in UK government workfare programmes. *Medical Humanities*. 41, pp.40–47.

Greenberg, G. (2011) The failure of biogenetic analysis in psychology: Why psychology is not a biological science. *Research in Human Development*. 8, pp.173–191.

Insell, T. (2013) *Director's blog: Transforming diagnosis*, April 29, 2013. Available from: www.nimh.nih.gov/about/director/2013/transforming-diagnosis.shtml [Accessed 10 November 2016].

Kendler, K. S. (2016) The nature of psychiatric disorders. *World Psychiatry*. 15, pp.5–12.

Kubie, L. S. (1974) The myths of Thomas Szasz. *Bulletin of the Menninger Clinic*. 38, pp.497–502.

Leifer, R. (2016) *On the psychiatric repression of Thomas Szasz: Its social and political significance*. Available from: www.psychotherapy.net [Accessed 10 March 2016].

Leifer, R. (1990) The medical model as the ideology of the therapeutic state. *Journal of Mind and Behavior*. 11(3–4), pp.247–258.

Lilienfeld, S. O. & Marino, L. (1995) Mental disorder as a Roschian concept: A critique of Wakefield's "harmful dysfunction" analysis. *Journal of Abnormal Psychology*. 104(3), pp.411–420.

Marková, I. S. & Berrios, G. E. (2016) Research in psychiatry: Concepts and conceptual analysis. *Psychopathology*. 49, pp.188–194.

Martin, R. & Barresi, J. (2006) *The rise and fall of soul and self: An intellectual history of personal identity*. New York, Columbia University Press.
Moncrieff. J. (2014) 'Freedom is more important than health': Thomas Szasz and the problem of paternalism. *International Psychiatry*. 11, pp.4–8.
Papineau, D. (1994) Mental disorder, illness and biological disfunction. *Philosophy*. 37, pp.73–82.
Paris, J. & Kirmeyer, L. J. (2016) The National Institute of Mental Health research domain criteria: A bridge too far. *Journal of Nervous and Mental Disease*. 204, pp.26–32.
Peters, R. S. (1967) *The concept of motivation*. London, Routledge & Kegan Paul.
Pickering, N. (2006) *The metaphor of mental illness*. Oxford, Oxford University Press.
Pies. R. (1979) On myths and countermyths, *Archives of General Psychiatry*. 26, pp.139–44.
Pols, J. (2005). *The politics of mental illness: Myth and power in the work of Thomas S. Szasz*, trans. from Dutch by Mira de Vries. Available from: www.janpols.net/Pols-PDF.pdf [Accessed 10 March 2017].
Sedgwick, P. (1982) *Psycho politics*. London, Pluto Press.
Sedgwick, P. (1972) Mental illness is illness. *Salmagundi*. 20, pp.196–224.
Smith, R. (1992) *Inhibition: History and meaning in the sciences of mind and brain*. Berkeley, CA, University of California Press.
Szasz, T. (2011) The myth of mental illness: 50 years later. *The Psychiatrist*. 35, pp.179–182.
Szasz, T. (2010 [1961]) *The myth of mental illness: Foundations of a theory of personal conduct*. New York, Harper Perennial.
Szasz, T. (2007) *The medicalization of everyday life*. New York, Syracuse University Press.
Szasz, T. (2003) The cure of souls in the therapeutic state. *The Psychoanalytic Review*. 90, pp.45–62.
Szasz, T. (1988 [1978]) Persuading persons: Rhetoric as remedy. In: T. Szasz (ed.) *The myth of psychotherapy*. Syracuse, NY, Syracuse University Press, pp.11–24.
Szasz, T. (1984) *The therapeutic state*. New York, Prometheus Books.
Vice, J. (1993) *From patients to persons: The psychiatric critiques of Thomas Szasz, Peter Sedgwick, and R. D. Laing*. New York, Peter Lang.
Wakefield, J. C. (1992) Disorder as harmful dysfunction: A conceptual critique of DSM-III-R's definition of mental disorder. *Psychological Review*. 99, pp.232–247.
Young, J. T. (2004) Illness behavior: A selective review and synthesis. *Sociology of Health and Illness*. 26, pp.1–31.
Zupan, M. L. (1973) Is mental illness a myth? *Reason*, 5, p.3.

3

'MENTAL' AND 'BODILY' CAUSES OF WOES

A brief history

The word 'mental' in 'mental illness' is obviously intended to differentiate it from physical illness. In this chapter, I discuss early accounts of the causes of woes and briefly trace the developments that led to the contemporary division of illness into mental and physical categories. I relate this division to two types of explanation, namely mechanism and contextualism, and contrast them using historical illustrations and contemporary psychiatric diagnosis. I end with a section that sets out a schematic framework for integrating somatic (bodily) type explanations with psychosocial (mental) accounts of the causes of woes.

Mind and body: historical antecedents

The modern idea that a woe is related to, or caused by, something occurring in a person's mind or body is not one with easily traceable historical roots. We have little to go on when speculating about how mind and body were distinguished, if at all, before this question was ever discussed in written form. It is possible that things we regard as 'mental' (e.g. experience and knowledge) rather than 'material' (e.g. objects and bodies) were not distinguished by our forebears. The distinction between mind and body remains contentious even in present scientific debates. For instance, in research on the abilities of the higher primates, it has been asked whether an animal can attribute a 'mental state' to another member of its own social group (Penn and Povinelli, 2009). Some theorists feel that it is unnecessary to introduce the concept of mental states and they interpret social interaction between animals in terms of animals responding to one another's concrete behaviour, that is, simply using it as a cue to their own future behaviour. In sum, we do not yet know how the signs for mind, body, or even individual identity, evolved biologically and culturally. It is possible that for tens of thousands of years, human experience was not seen as being caused by, or existing within, a separately identified mind and body.

Concepts that we now associate with mind and body are found in the earliest recorded mytho-philosophical schemes for explaining the world. Historians, philosophers, and anthropologists have long assumed that one way to interpret ancient literature, and pre-literate cultures more generally, is through their employment of figurative language. That is, simile, analogy, metaphor, and metonymy have been seen as means that people have used to grasp complex phenomena. That which is unfamiliar or unknown is assimilated into the familiar (e.g. Cazeneuve, 1972: 14).

Classical Greece

The cosmologies of the ancient Greeks sought answers to metaphysical questions through reference to fire, water, earth, and air. The word for soul (*psyche*) was derived from the word for breath. *Thymos* was associated with breath and blood, and was assumed by Plato to be a constituent element of *psyche*, namely spiritedness, passion, or desire. The phenomenon of breathing is experienced visibly as well as being felt and heard, and it can be seen to stop, sometimes with loud vocalisations, when a person dies. It is perhaps not surprising that breathing was related to abstract notions of life, death, and immortality. There are many examples in ancient literature of 'unknown' (i.e. hidden and speculative) causes being understood by linking them directly to the experienced world. Democritus (c.460–c.370 BC) could extend the perceptible quality of smallness to imagine the world composed of infinitely small particles or atoms. Atoms could take different shapes; soul atoms (also of a material nature) differed from other atoms in being more subtle and rapid in motion (Peters, 1962: 47–51).

Hippocrates (c.460–c.370 BC) founded a school of medicine that was important in displacing a belief in occult and demonic causes of woes. Hippocrates also contributed greatly by describing in considerable detail the physical signs of different illnesses and producing a system for classifying them. He did not entirely dispense with the supernatural because he still believed that signs of divine influence could be read into dreams (Peters, 1962: 59). However, his view of the cause of what is now called mental illness was essentially somatic; it 'arises from a humid condition of the brain which causes it to move perpetually and produce confusion of the senses' (ibid.: 58).

The belief that so-called mental illness has a neural basis can therefore be traced back to ancient somatic theories about the material state of the brain. However, Hippocrates' theory of the causes of a state of health, and the role of the brain within it, hardly resembles any modern theory at all. His account of health was not confined to the body because it included the climate, the seasons, the locality, the winds, and the stars. Air, fire, and water were central concepts. The brain was no more than a medium through which 'air' communicated its nature to us. Hippocrates' theory was therefore primarily environmental, and his remedies stressed the importance of exercise and diet. The Hippocratic account of illness (both 'physical' or 'mental') drew upon earlier ideas about certain bodily fluids (the four humours) thought to affect human personality traits and behaviour. Bell (2014: 39), a historian, notes that Hippocrates did not treat these substances as instances of pathophysiology. Humors were normal substances, and ill-health was explained by a lack of balance between them. Hippocrates' theory therefore integrated what we would now consider to be the 'mental', the 'physical', and the 'environmental' in a way that does not resemble any contemporary biomedical theory.

Bell (2014: 40) suggests that a disease concept of 'melancholy' pre-dated humoral theory (ibid.: 64). He points out that the main remedies were physical, such as purging. Bell concludes that there is a cluster of woes that have been described for at least two and half thousand years that we can safely interpret as a psychiatric disorder. Bell's position (ibid.: 9) is that melancholy is a 'natural kind' (i.e. a bodily pathology) although he thinks its expression can be modified by social and cultural circumstances:

> Melancholia could become prominent and widely used only when a realist mental medicine and a culture of self-consciousness had become embedded in fifth century BC Greece, and that melancholia's continuing prominence within Western culture and latterly the spread of depression to many parts of the world depends on these same vectors.
>
> *Bell, 2014: 23*

This is a good historical summing up but not, of course, currently a sound basis for drawing any conclusions about melancholy or depression as an illness or psychiatric disorder.

A different tradition in ancient Greece, addressing itself to a person's well-being, can be found in the writings of Plato and Aristotle (Irwin, 2015). This tradition is concerned with the state of the soul, and therefore, in modern terms it advocated a moral or psychological approach to madness or distress. In essence, Plato and Aristotle focused on the element of a lack of control by the soul (and especially the soul's faculty of 'reason'), with an effect that leads to the soul being usurped by the appetites or passions. By this means, these two philosophers imagined that the soul lost its moral qualities of unity and virtue. According to Plato, a person's reason had to arbitrate on behalf of the whole soul, and a person 'has to be a friend to him/herself'. The concept of soul later became the concept of mind, and the battle between reason and passion has had echoes in theories throughout the centuries.

From ancient to early modern views: Robert Burton (1621)

Burton's description and explanation of the condition he called melancholy (Burton, 2001) are interesting because, as a librarian at Christ Church College, Oxford, he had access to a wealth of ancient literature and quoted from his sources at length (Nicol, 1948). Burton was writing before the birth of Isaac Newton (in 1642) and seems to have had one foot in the ancient world and one in the contemporary. While Burton was very open-minded and expatiated on many ideas, however fanciful, behind this facade lay a common-sense and logical mind. He foresaw a National Health Service publicly provided for all those in need of it: 'Hospitals of all kinds, for children, orphans, old folks, sick men, mad men, soldiers, pest houses, etc., not built precario [i.e. only to last a short time] or by gouty benefactors' (ibid.: 201).

Mirroring later contests between the medical profession and its competitors in the field of human woes, Burton had to doff his cap to physicians (humorously, it must be said) before he set out his own opinions:

> If any physician in the meantime shall infer, *Ne sutor ultra crepidam*, and find himself grieved that I have intruded into his profession, I will tell him in brief, I do not otherwise by them than they do by us, if it be for their advantage. I know many of their sect which have taken orders in hope of a benefice.
>
> *Burton, 2001: 36*

Burton's Latin expression means literally 'Shoemaker, not beyond the shoe', used to warn people to avoid passing judgement beyond their expertise.

Reading his ancient sources, it must have been very difficult for Burton to differentiate the relative importance of causes in the body, in the physical environment, and in a person's social circumstances. In fact, Burton does not attempt to do so and covers everything as of potentially equal importance. As he puts it:

> It is a disease of the soul in which I am to treat and as much appertaining to a Divine as to a Physician. A good divine either is or ought to be a good physician – a spiritual physician at least. They differ but in object, the one of the body, the other of the soul, and use divers medicines to cure.
>
> *Nicol, 1948: 201*

Burton believed that the causes of the so-called mental illnesses of his day rested on opinion, whereas the causes of bodily disease were more obvious. He was wise to the need for proof when it came to attributing melancholy to a malfunctioning body. He reasoned that the widely supposed bodily cause of melancholy (an excess of 'black bile') could just as well be a consequence of the malady as its cause:

> The name is imposed from the matter, and disease denominated from the material cause, from black choler. And whether it be a cause or an effect, a disease or a symptom, let Donatus Altomarus and Salvanius decide; I will not contend about it.
>
> *Burton 2001: 169*

Burton produced elaborate classifications for the nature, causes, and cures of melancholy. He distinguished madness (e.g. violent, angry, ravings without fear or sorrow) from melancholy proper, and states of melancholy. Melancholy could come and go (rather like a habit), was not associated with fever, and was accompanied by fear and sadness for which there was no apparent occasion. He also noted it could lead to suicide (Nicol, 1948: 202). According to Burton, the causes of melancholy were so diverse that no one of them could be considered as the main one. He mentioned sin, the stars, heredity, diet, sexual abstinence, sexual obsession, over-indulgence, violent exercise, idleness, shame, and excessive studying. The list of potential cures was equally long, although he deplored witchcraft, sorcery, magic, and quack empirics who 'to get a fee, will give Physick to everyone that comes, when there is no cause' (ibid.: 204). He proposed three main forms of therapy: 'Diet or Living' (e.g. outdoor exercise, recreations for the mind), 'Apothecary' (e.g. the herbs borage and bugloss, and purgatives such as hellebore and tobacco), and 'Chirurgery' (e.g. leeches, blood letting, and boring into the skull). Burton was not enthusiastic about physical remedies, writing that 'Physicians kill as many as they save, and who can tell how many murders they make in a year, that may freely kill folks, and have a reward for it?' (ibid.)

It is widely supposed that Burton suffered from melancholy himself because he says as much. Given the wide compass of his ideas, it is not surprising that he insisted on an accurate assessment: '. . . be not too niggardly miserable of the purse or think it too much that he bestows upon himself, and to save charges endanger his health' (Nicol, 1948: 204). It is notable that although Burton distinguished between mental and bodily illness, he was open to entertaining almost any conceivable cause of these conditions.

In the century that followed Burton, the somatic, dietary, and other medical explanations for what today would be seen as woes of a primarily psychosocial nature continued to be popular (Porter, 1987; Newton, 2013: 123). Porter argues that a treatment focused on the body was useful to ordinary people because it was what they wished to believe, serving to cover up the actual sources of their woes, which, if revealed, could lead to dishonour, guilt, or reproach.

Current concepts of 'the mental' seem to be no less metaphorical than they were for the ancient Greeks. The concept of mind cannot be defined in a way that would satisfy most natural scientists. Gilbert Ryle (1949) famously called it the 'ghost in the machine'. Mind is imagined as a virtual space with no obvious boundaries (except that it happens to belong to an individual person). It contains 'mental events' that succeed each other in time (but the events cannot easily be identified separately or given a precise duration). Mental characteristics usually have to be communicated retrospectively by proxy – in other words, by referring to a shared public sign, such as a word or phrase, a cross on a rating scale, or by comparison with a sensation. The symptoms that define so-called mental illness also rely on figurative language. The concept of 'self', as in 'low self-esteem' is not something that can be given an empirical status. It has been compared to a virtual object or avatar, serving as a short cut to saying something far more complex that is appreciated only intuitively (Hallam, 2009). We have a notion of what is meant by 'low self-esteem' but any interviewer assessing someone who complains of it would want to be provided with examples and ask for the where, when, how, and why of this complaint. In the abstract, and labelled as a symptom, it lacks concrete meaning.

Discussion of a person's self usually leads to a wider exploration of a person's hopes, values, ambitions, regrets, and disappointments. In past eras, this kind of discourse might have been understood as a reflection on the state of a person's soul. Although we now rarely use this terminology, the word 'soulless' still resonates with meaning, whether applied to persons or places. The concept of mind came about as a gradual transformation of the concept of soul in the early modern period (Martin and Barresi, 2006). The transformation from soul to mind took place at a time when people began to adopt a rational and secular outlook, and when materialistic interpretations of the natural world were rapidly gaining ground. The materialist trajectory eventually led to an understanding of the mind as a machine, and mind was equated with the functioning of the brain. This narrow view of the cause of all things 'mental' is unconvincing. We may have to revert back to a concept of mind that resonates more closely with the concept of soul. The idea of recovering one's soul might sound quaint. If this perspective takes hold, recovery from so-called mental illness will no longer be seen as a process of correcting a dysfunctional body.

Mechanism versus contextualism

The idea that a person's belief in a somatic cause of their woes can serve a psychosocial function is implied by the contemporary psychiatric concept of 'somatisation'. A person might worry excessively about pain, fatigue, or weakness, believing them to be a sign of serious disease, and spend much time and energy having them medically investigated. Although a person who presents in this way is called 'disordered', the role of any disorder of the body is obscure. The existence of 'somatisation' (and other psychiatric categories) reflects the employment of two competing modes of explanation: mechanism (e.g. bodily mechanics) and contextualism (e.g. contextual influences of a psychosocial kind that serve an explanatory function) (Pepper, 1942; Hayes, Hayes and Reese, 1988).

In ancient Greece, Hippocrates' emphasis on empirical observation and the classification of illnesses (based on a mechanistic model) was in striking contrast with an older tradition that woes could be explained by the malevolent intentions of a god (a contextual account). According to the classicist Fontaigne (2013), Hippocratic ideas competed with the usual remedy for displeasing a god, which was to make an animal sacrifice. Fontaigne maintains that Hippocrates' medical approach was parodied early on in a Greek comedy that was later adapted by the Roman playwright Paulanus. The comedy shows how an identical twin's frustrated reaction to being mistaken for his own twin is misinterpreted by his family and their physician as a sign of insanity. In other words, like a modern psychiatrist consulting a diagnostic manual, the physician ignores the circumstances in which a normal human reaction can be understood (for the audience, this is clearly given by the play's plot), checks off symptoms listed in the manual, and diagnoses a disorder of the mind. The protesting patient is led away to an institution. This was and still is a parody of what happens, but it can get uncomfortably close to the truth.

The point of the play is that apparently inexplicable conduct can be explained contextually. Unknown to the family and their physician, the protagonist's long-lost identical twin brother had unexpectedly visited the town, and the inhabitants, including the protagonist's mistress, had greeted him with open arms (and legs). The ravings of the other twin's anger were mistaken for the ravings of a madman, but on this occasion they were quite understandable once the circumstances were known. In order to appreciate the play, it is necessary to switch between a mechanistic and contextual explanation.

The root metaphor of mechanism is the machine, in which the individual parts are systematically related to each other, so that together, with an appropriate transmission of force through the system, a predictable outcome results. Some systems of the body seem to work in this way. At night, while asleep, the body ticks over without any obvious supervening influence. When awake, we can speed up and slow down our breathing, but by and large, when we are asleep the system operates automatically with homeostatic adjustments when the body needs more or less oxygen. All parts of a machine should ideally work together in harmony and so, in the case of so-called mental illness, it is concluded that one part (known or unknown) is malfunctioning. It is assumed that mental processes correspond to neural processes, and so the brain is usually equated with the boundaries of the machine.

The motive lying behind the creation of a mental illness is to model it on physical illness. For instance, the problem becomes a list of symptoms, and clues to their contextual understanding are removed. An example from the *Diagnostic and statistical manual of mental disorders: DSM-5* is 'persistent difficulty discarding or parting with possessions' (DSM, 2013). Hoarding is not, at first sight, a disorder of any bodily mechanism but, rather, is a description of a person going about their business in an unusual way. To call it a symptom is to compare it with a spot on the skin which a doctor might be examining for its potentially sinister implications. A failure to discard apparently worthless possessions can certainly exceed reasonable limits but to describe it as a symptom, without saying what it is a symptom of, does not go beyond describing the way things are or appear. It is like a spot on the skin which, so far, it has not been possible to explain as a sign of something else. The degree of hoarding may be disabling and the person him or herself may experience it as compulsive. The strength of the habit might stretch the bounds of everyday explanation. When viewed medically, it is classified as a disorder and this designation may initiate a search for biological signs of a disordered somatic process.

In brief, psychiatric disorders are defined by decontextualised phenomena that people seem willing to have explained medically. The disorder explanation is attractive because it satisfies our curiosity when normal assumptions about the causes of behaviour have been violated. Most people do not hoard personal possessions to the point that they can barely walk across a room. So-called symptoms might feel like illness because they are unbidden, out of our control, and debilitating. However, this does not mean that an explanation in terms of physiological processes or structural defects in the body is required or appropriate. It is true that hoarding could not take place without neurophysiological responses to sensory stimuli, but this may not be the level to seek for an explanation or effect a change. Hoarding is essentially a form of behaviour, and it is a problem because society (or the woeful individual) regards it as such.

In contrast to mechanism, a contextual explanation makes reference to the quality of experience, and the surrounding circumstances and relations that contribute to that quality (Hayes et al., 1988). An adequate description of an act therefore has to spread out to whatever is relevant in this respect. For instance, the context of receiving a reward might be relevant, such as who is delivering it, in what manner, and how the reward is spread out in space and time. From a contextual perspective, the boundaries of the analysis are determined by what the analysis sets out to achieve – in other words, its goals. The success of this approach is determined by pragmatic criteria. For instance, if a person presents with the problem of an extreme fear of spiders, and wishes to overcome it, we could ask whether it is necessary to go beyond analysing the size and species of the offending spider or consider whether other circumstances are relevant as well. For many so-called mental illnesses, a therapist's assessment of a problem is likely to extend into the distant past and foreseeable future. The person who does the assessment is also a relevant thread in the analysis because she or he is also part of the context in which information is elicited, and therefore partly shapes its outcome.

The idea that an explanation of all things of a mental nature can be reduced to the brain and the employment of the machine metaphor has been called the mereological fallacy (Bennett and Hacker, 2003). By contrast, a contextual account of 'mind' includes persons because it is a person who acts, not a brain. The social practices in which a person participates depend on shared knowledge in a public form (a shared language, the written word, codified procedures, etc.). All of this information about the world is co-opted rather than stored in the mind or brain. In this sense, the mind is 'extended' into the outside world. The thesis of an 'extended mind' is not yet widely accepted, and it is evident from citations in the previous chapter that many philosophers and researchers continue to believe that, in the case of so-called mental illness, there is no need to look beyond the brain. For them, mental illness is brain illness.

Pandya (2011), a neurosurgeon, expresses commonly held assumptions when he traces ancient to modern thinking about the relationship between mind, brain, and soul. He concludes that the mind and soul remain fascinating enigmas but goes on to assert that 'the brain is the organ of the mind just as the lungs are the organs for respiration.' He also believes that we must continue to search for the soul's location. He quotes Prioreschi (1996), who translates an excerpt from a text of Hippocrates (from *On the sacred disease*) as follows: 'I hold that the brain is the most powerful organ of the human body . . . wherefore I assert that the brain is the interpreter of consciousness . . .'

Although, as I have already noted, Hippocrates implicated the brain in all sorts of phenomena, Brett's interpretation of Hippocratic writings about the role of the brain places it in a different light. According to Brett, air was the central concept for Hippocrates, and the brain mediated its distribution. The Hippocratic text translated above also refers to 'consciousness', but according to Müller-Freienfels, no word exists for consciousness in most languages. He argues that for the Greeks and Romans, it was not a fundamental antonym to the physical. In Plato and Aristotle, a great deal of what we call consciousness was ascribed to the body rather than the soul. A concept of conscious awareness as a property of mind or brain (the sense in which we typically employ the term) seems to depend on having a concept of being conscious of consciousness. Müller-Freienfels (1935: 36) considers this idea did not emerge until Descartes in the seventeenth century, when he drew a sharp distinction between mind substance and body substance.

An association between soul and material substance was maintained right up to Descartes in the seventeenth century, although he conceived of mind substance (or, as he referred to it, 'mind or soul') as being unchanging and indivisible. This content-less view of mind substance therefore left no room for a materialist analysis of the contents of the minds of different persons. However, Descartes added in the notion of mind substance interacting with the body substance of the brain, where abnormalities of various sorts were imagined to exist (López-Muñoz et al., 2011). The legacy of brain abnormalities has lived on ever since.

Some psychiatrists accept that the mechanistic metaphor of disorder can be over-extended (Horwitz and Wakefield, 2007: Chapter 3). These authors go part of the way in accepting a contextual explanation for depressed mood. They interpret ancient literature on melancholia as supporting a distinction between 'normal sadness' and depressed mood understood as an illness or disease. Their position is that so-called depressive illness is either a set of symptoms that cannot be explained contextually or the expression of a bodily constitution that is more than averagely predisposed to melancholy when confronted by the usual type of triggering events.

Horwitz and Wakefield cite examples from classical literature in which what appeared to be the disease of melancholy was found subsequently to have an adequate contextual explanation. The support these authors seek for their position from classical literature therefore has to face two objections. First is the fact that the attribution of melancholy to a disease process may be as mistaken today as it was in the past. Second, if ancient physicians sometimes acknowledged mistaking normal sadness for melancholic disease, how do we know that physicians do not make a similar mistake today? A depressed mood that is intense and seems disproportionate to circumstances could turn out to be a condition whose contextual causes have not been adequately investigated. The causes could be undetected distal events of a psychosocial nature. In any case, mechanistic and contextual explanations are not mutually exclusive. Even granted that there may be important somatic causes that contribute to depressed mood (genetic predisposition, dysfunctions, physical illness, etc.), the context in which these causes arise can still be highly relevant and influential. For this reason, either/or debates about the causes of woes can prove fruitless when the interaction between somatic and psychosocial factors is unknown and likely to be complex.

The machine model of mind encounters several problems. One obvious difficulty when literally equating mind with body is that mental experience bears no resemblance whatsoever to neural tissue and a person can function normally without knowing whether or he or she even possesses a brain. There are, of course, correspondences between mental experiences and events in the brain, as shown by stimulating it directly or imaging the brain's activity with scanning techniques. There is an assumed and undoubted connection between experiences and neural events but no consensus on how the relationship should be understood. Controversy has been stirred up by experiments showing that neural events associated with a person deciding to flick their wrist precede an awareness of having made a freely willed decision to do so (Libet, 2000). It is as if a person's brain has already made up the person's mind for them – that a neural cause has preceded the mental event of willing something to happen. This has given grounds for believing that the mind is simply a reflection of neural events.

However, this interpretation of the experimental findings decontextualises the experiment and erroneously supports an inappropriate adoption of the machine model. Put simply, it is a person, not a brain, who has been asked to flick their wrist at a self-chosen signal. And it is a person, not a brain, who responds to the consequences of their actions, discovering whether or not their willed action has yielded its expected consequence. It is quite conceivable that knowledge of consequences (which therefore implicates conscious decision making) can act retrospectively on a preceding neural process in so far as it influences how this cause functions on future occasions. This remains a deterministic theory but it recognises that there is a causal role for all of the environmental and cultural determinants of conscious thought.

The brain does of course control many habitual actions without a person's awareness or conscious monitoring of the consequences of an act. However, the existence of a monitoring function becomes obvious when the consequences (even of an automatic habit) are unexpected. For instance, a person may become alarmed by a feeling that 'they cannot breathe', when, in reality, a shutting down of their respiratory muscles is likely to have been the body's homeostatic response to over-breathing. By breathing too rapidly or deeply, a person can disturb the balance between oxygen and carbon dioxide concentrations in the blood, this being one signal for a homeostatic mechanism to correct this state of affairs. Respiration is shut down and a person experiences this as being 'unable to get their breath'.

Learning takes place when the consequences of an event influence a person's subsequent response to that event (or a similar one) on future occasions. In the example just provided, the person worries that they will continue to have a breathing problem, or worse still, that they are suffering from a cardiovascular condition; they then become alerted to any signal that this could be true. Behavioural psychologists refer to consequences that strengthen a behaviour as 'rewards' and those that weaken it, 'punishments'. Brains mediate behaviour but they do not reward or punish themselves. A person may arrange for a reward or punishment to follow an act (performed by someone else or one that they perform themselves) but in this case it is a person deciding to do so in response to other influences, and not the brain 'of its own accord'. If one wished to pursue the machine metaphor, the boundaries of the machine would have to extend outside the brain and include the environment. This move towards 'supersizing the mind' (the title of a book by philosopher Andrew Clark, 2008) leads us into questioning the traditionally understood boundaries between mind and body.

A schematic framework for 'mental' and 'bodily' explanations

I assume that explanations of behaviour can be formulated at different levels of analysis, from the most fundamental physical-particle level to the most inclusive sociological, political, and historical levels (Hallam, 2009: 267). I also assume that there is upward and downward causation between events that are understood at higher and lower levels of explanation. For instance, a fearful response to driving after a road traffic accident could be changed by imbibing alcohol (upward causation from the somatic level on the elicitation of fear), or by reappraising the risks and gradually overcoming fear by a gradual reintroduction to the experience of driving (downward causation from the psychological level on the mediation of fear at a somatic level).

Another relevant distinction, introduced in earlier chapters, is between distal and proximal causes of a woe. The distal causes are all past events, at all levels of analysis, that have influenced the current expression of a woe. The proximal causes are all present events (at all levels of analysis) that are sufficient to bring it about. The distal causes of a woe can be conceptualised at several levels, singly or in combination (genetic, somatic, psychosocial, cultural, etc.), but the proximal causes are usually distinguishable with less ambiguity. A physical illness is typically identifiable as a characteristic malfunction or impairment, having proximal causes in some part or system of the body. This is rarely the case with a so-called mental illness. The hoarder, in other words, may pass any medical assessment of the state of their physical health. In effect, I assume that for most woes, it is possible to make a reasonable guess about the nature of the *primary proximal* cause. It would be obvious, say, in the case of exposure to an infectious agent versus exposure to a psychologically traumatising event, such as a road traffic accident, that did not cause injury to the body. However, the distal causes would be far more difficult to identify – that is, why a person might have been susceptible to infection or why they reacted to an accident with greater or lesser psychological distress.

One practical test for differentiating between the proximal causes of so-called physical and mental illnesses is whether the woe could potentially be resolved by modifying the influence of noxious psychosocial causes, past or present. For instance, in the case of hoarding, could the habit be changed by a method based on re-learning? A failure to pass this test would not prove the presence of a proximal cause having the nature of a somatic dysfunction, but passing it makes it much less likely. In some cases, success is more likely to be achieved by combining a psychosocial with a somatic intervention, such as a medication. If this proved to be the case for hoarding, it would not be safe to conclude that the problem should be attributed to the existence of a somatic dysfunction. This hypothesis cannot be ruled out, but it would require a theoretical rationale and additional empirical support to be convincing.

The position of many biomedical psychiatrists is that there is no need to distinguish between mental and physical illness as far as causation is concerned. Kendell argues that 'the distinction between mental and physical illness is unfounded and incompatible with contemporary understanding of disease.' He reaches this conclusion by pointing out that for over two thousand years physicians have treated conditions 'that would now be regarded as mental illnesses' with the same interventions they offered for more obviously physical complaints. This is certainly a historical fact but why they did so is not relevant to the question of a correct view of causation today. Kendell dates the origins of the concept of mental illness to the end of the eighteenth century, when moral treatment was found to be effective in curing insanity, even though the approach was not a medical one. It was introduced into the newly built asylums that eventually came to be managed by physicians who continued the long tradition of regarding the body as the seat of all problems. However, as a somatic cause could not be found for most forms of insanity, the conditions they treated were regarded as 'psychogenic' or 'functional' illnesses. Kendell believes that this was an unfortunate development because, for him, 'all thinking physicians' know that mental disorders 'are not fundamentally different from other illnesses' (2001: 490–493).

Kendell argues that 'psyche' and 'soma' are involved in all illness. Pain and depressed mood are 'psychological' phenomena, and 'emotions' can cause bodily illness. All of the foregoing is unquestionably true but beside the point. Psychological phenomena and emotions are not usually understood and influenced in the same way that bodily dysfunctions are explained and treated by physicians. Non-medical experts are called in because medical knowledge does not provide a basis for psychosocial therapy. The fact that psychiatrists happen to be medically trained and are continuing an ancient tradition (and are now managing mental health facilities) has no bearing on the issue of causation.

Kendell rests his case on the fact that there is 'unassailable evidence' that 'somatic abnormalities' are involved in 'depressive illness' and many other 'illnesses' that he mentions. These claims are essential if psychiatry is to justify its professional position. Of course, if demonstrable pathology can be discovered, that is all well and good (see Chapter 4). However, the evidence for somatic pathology (as distinct from somatic processes that are not pathological) is very thin on the ground. In the case of genetic evidence, we are usually dealing with a risk factor, something that predisposes a person to develop a so-called mental illness. A genetic predisposition is not pathology as such, except in rare cases. Predispositions exist for nearly all forms of behaviour, good or bad, and they are only worth knowing about if they have treatment implications, which in large measure they do not.

In Kendell's opinion, mental and physical illnesses are indistinguishable in terms of aetiology or symptomatology. He points out that disease caused by psychosocial factors (e.g. emotional events that precipitate a myocardial infarction) shows that there is no difference between the causes of so-called mental and physical illness. This deduction is illogical. It merely shows that an interaction between events conceptualised at different levels of analysis can have pathological consequences. When emotional states cause cardiac disease, we can distinguish this situation from others where emotional states do not cause disease. Emotional states, per se, are not the cause of illness, mental or physical. In those situations in which psychosocial events appear to be adequate to account for so-called mental illness, there is no reason to compare the latter with a physical illness. It is unquestionably of great interest to know how events at the psychosocial level relate to the biological level, and hopefully, causal mechanisms will be elucidated. This knowledge may or may not be relevant when attempts are made to alter a pathogenic emotional state.

A belief in the reality of 'mental illness' as disease has important implications for public attitudes and public policy. Kendell states that developing a 'mental illness' has nothing to do with 'a certain lack of moral fibre' or 'free will'. Presumably, the hoarder simply has to retire to bed and take their pill or injection. The idea that problems in living that are currently rendered as illnesses have nothing to do with a person's desire and motivation to change is inconsistent with both common sense and philosophical accounts of volition.

Summary

A brief review of ideas about mind and body in ancient literature shows that they differ substantially from current ways of differentiating mind and body. The early conceptions took in the nature of the cosmos, the state of the soul, and both social and environmental determinants. The later transformation of soul into mind, and the identification of mind with the brain, has meant that earlier connotations of soul and the wider context have been lost. Current attempts to discover the causes of so-called mental illness in the brain have not taken sufficient account of upward and downward causation between processes conceptualised at different levels of analysis. Decontextualised definitions of symptoms and disorders do not integrate distal determining influences on woes with a person's construction of past, present, and future. Attempts to reduce the causes of so-called 'mental illness' to a biological level are narrow and unconvincing.

References

Bell, M. (2014) *Melancholia: The Western malady*. Cambridge, Cambridge University Press.

Bennett, M. R. & Hacker. P. (2003) *Philosophical foundations of neuroscience*. Oxford, Blackwell.

Burton, R. (2001) *The anatomy of melancholy*. New York, New York Review of Books.

Cazeneuve, J. (1972) *Lucien Levy-Bruhl*. Trans. Riviere, P. Oxford, Blackwell.

Clark, A. (2008) *Supersizing the mind: Embodiment, action, and cognitive extension*. Oxford, Oxford University Press.

DSM (2013) *Diagnostic and statistical manual of mental disorders: DSM-5*. Washington, DC, American Psychiatric Association.

Fontaigne, M. (2013) On being sane in an insane place – The Rosenhan experiment in the laboratory of Plautus' Epidamnus. *Current Psychology*. 32, p.348.

Hallam, R. S. (2009) *Virtual selves, real persons: A dialogue across disciplines*. Cambridge, Cambridge University Press.

Hayes, S. C., Hayes, L. J. & Reese, H. W. (1988) Finding the philosophical core: A review of Stephen C. Pepper's *World hypotheses: A study in evidence*. *Journal of the Experimental Analysis of Behavior*. 50, pp.97–111.

Horwitz, A. V. & Wakefield, J. C. (2007) *The loss of sadness: How psychiatry transformed normal sorrow into depressive disorder*. New York, Oxford University Press.

Irwin, T. H. (2015) Mental health as moral virtue: Some ancient arguments. In: Fulford, K. W. M. et al. (eds.) *The Oxford handbook of philosophy and psychiatry*. Oxford, Oxford University Press, pp.47–52.

Kendell, R. E. (2001) The distinction between mental and physical illness. *British Journal of Psychiatry*. 178(6), pp.490–493.

Libet, B. (2000) Do we have free will? In: Libet, B., Freeman, A. & Sutherland, K. (eds.) *The volitional brain: Towards a neuroscience of free will*. Exeter, Imprint Academic, pp.47–58.

López-Muñoz, F., Rubio, G., Molina, J. D. & Alamo, C. (2011) Sadness as a passion of the soul: A psychopathological consideration of the Cartesian concept of melancholy. *Brain Research Bulletin*. 85, pp.42–53.

Martin, R. & Barresi, J. (2006) *The rise and fall of soul and self: An intellectual history of personal identity*. New York, Columbia University Press.

Müller-Freienfels, R. (1935) *The evolution of modern psychology*, trans. Wolfe, W. B. New Haven, CT, Yale University Press.

Newton, J. (2013) *Preventing mental ill-health: Informing public health planning and mental health practice*. London, Routledge.

Nicol, W. D. (1948) Robert Burton's *Anatomy of Melancholy*. *Postgraduate Medical Journal*. 24(270), pp.199–206.

Pandya, S. K. (2011) Understanding brain, mind and soul: Contributions from neurology and neurosurgery. In: Singh, A. R. & Singh S. A. (eds.) *Brain, mind and consciousness: An international, interdisciplinary perspective*. *MSM*, 9(1), pp.129–149. Available at www.msmonographs.org/article.asp?issn=0973-1229;year=2011;volume=9;issue=1;spage=129;epage=149;aulast=Pandya [Accessed 10 December 2017].

Penn, D. C. & Povinelli. D. J. (2009) On becoming approximately rational: The relational reinterpretation hypothesis. In Watanabe, A. P. et al. (eds.) *Rational animals, irrational humans*. Tokyo, Keio University Press.

Pepper, S. C. (1942) *World hypotheses: A study of evidence*. Berkeley, CA, University of California Press.

Peters, R. S. (1962) *Brett's history of psychology*, ed. and abridged. London, George, Allen & Unwin.

Porter, R. (1987) *Mind forg'd manacles: Madness and psychiatry in England from the Restoration to Regency*. London, Athlone.

Prioreschi, P. (1996) *A history of medicine: Greek Medicine. Vol. 2*. Omaha, NE, Horatius Press.

Ryle, G. (1949) *The concept of mind*. London, Hutchinson.

4

'MAJOR DEPRESSION'

The creation of a mythical disease

Depressed mood is an unremarkable and familiar human experience and so its formulation as an illness or disease has to be justified. One simple answer is to fall back on criteria for severity and persistence of the mood. It does not seem inappropriate to entertain a concept of pathology when the extreme can include self-starvation, bodily malfunction, and suicide. However, to take a disease hypothesis seriously, it is necessary to be sure that the set of behaviours typical of extreme mood can be reliably identified as medical syndromes. Researchers often lament that the population they are studying is heterogeneous, and they seek ways of identifying meaningful sub-groups. Unless variability in the way 'depression' presents itself can be assessed and understood, the results of research are likely to be inconclusive. Assessment relies heavily on questionnaires or standardised interviews that closely follow the model provided by psychiatric criteria. Research conducted to date does not inspire confidence that meaningful clinical syndromes have been identified.

Evidence for a disease perspective on the extremes of mood comes mainly from genetic studies and research into pathophysiology. After reviewing this evidence, the next section considers whether depressed mood is related to early experience, material and social circumstances, and gender. If it can be shown that variation in mood is chiefly related to social and environmental factors, support for a disease concept is lessened. It is, of course, necessary to research mood from all angles, and the extremes are likely to be a complex function of biological, psychological, and social variables acting together.

Psychiatric criteria for depressed/elated mood

If depression is a disease, one would expect to find (1) a cluster of signs and symptoms that can be reliably observed, and (2) an explanation of the cluster in terms of causal pathways discoverable within the body that are in some way distinct from the somatic correlates of everyday depressed mood. So far, this evidence is lacking and so it is implausible for the World Health Organization to claim that depression is a disease entity that ranks as 'the leading cause of disability worldwide' (WHO, 2015). In surveys of disease, depression is listed as not far behind cardiovascular disease and HIV/AIDS (Moussavi et al., 2007). It is projected that by 2030, depression will be ranked in the top three causes of 'disease burden' (Mathers and Loncar, 2006).

Leaving aside the problem of definition, the WHO does not always write about depression as if it were a disease. Many of the remedies it recommends on its website are unlike any treatment of a physical illness. It lists behavioural activation, cognitive behavioural therapy, and interpersonal psychotherapy before mentioning antidepressant medication. It advises that medication should not be the first line of treatment for mild depression (WHO, 2015). The implication seems to be that 'mild depression' is seen as an understandable reaction to adverse events, social situations, or psychological problems. Antidepressant medications have, of course, been marketed as treatment for a disease, often on the basis of spurious causal theories (Lynch, 2015). Many general physicians ignore WHO advice and prescribe medication as their first line of treatment for mild depression. They may not do this because they think depression is a disease but because there is a lengthy wait for alternative interventions, which may, in any case, be unavailable or unaffordable.

The WHO is charged with counting out the amount of ill-health and disability world-wide, and it has not unreasonably adopted pragmatic criteria for this purpose. However, the methods used for gathering data about 'depression' do not warrant the conclusion that there exists a biomedical disease causing almost as much 'burden' as cardiovascular disease or HIV/AIDS. This is not to say that severely depressed mood is not disabling. Mental health professionals use the term 'clinical depression' to distinguish a severe disturbance of mood from the temporary ups and downs that could be considered to lie within normal variation. Severity is indicated by a noticeable effect on areas of functioning such as appetite, sleep, mental concentration, self-worth, optimism, and sexual interest. The term 'clinical depression' means, in effect, that the alteration in mood is sufficiently extreme, enduring, and handicapping to warrant professional attention and support. However, it has proved extremely difficult to devise a set of criteria that clearly demarcate a clinical entity (or entities) centred on mood within the very broad spectrum of characteristics that make up normal variation. Criteria for a diagnosis of depression are not uniform, or uniformly applicable, across cultures (Pilgrim and Bentall, 1999). This is a serious objection when making a claim for an underlying disease process. A key to new discoveries is accurate description, and without it research flounders. With respect to depression, there is a degree of ambiguity and fluidity in diagnostic criteria that far exceeds the observational precision associated with the well-known physical diseases with which it has been compared.

The American Psychiatric Association's (APA) criteria for diagnosing 'major depressive disorder' (MDD) in *DSM-5* specify that a person must report one of two core symptoms and at least four of seven secondary symptoms (*DSM-5*, 2013). Some of these secondary symptoms are binary (e.g. insomnia or hypersomnia) and so the list effectively increases to twenty. In 3,703 individuals diagnosed according to these criteria, Fried and Nesse (2015) identified 1,030 unique symptom profiles. If the medical syndrome that supposedly links all these symptoms together is a fiction, a unitary concept of depression might as well be dispensed with altogether (Fried, 2016).

The psychological and behavioural phenomena that count as symptoms lie on continua, and so establishing that a symptom is present depends on exceeding a threshold of severity. Although there are guidelines for making this decision, it is inevitable that the criteria are difficult to apply. Furthermore, it is relatively easy to meet the *DSM-5* criteria for MDD, which requires only that a person complains of the necessary number of symptoms for a period of two weeks. Given this low threshold, it is not surprising to discover that MDD comes in grades of mild, moderate, and severe. In order to make sure that nothing has been missed, two other disorders have been invented: 'other specified depressive disorder' is reserved for people who do not meet full criteria for major depression, and 'unspecified depressive disorder' captures those people who do not meet full criteria for any kind of depressive disorder but there is insufficient evidence to state why. Adhering to these definitions, it is difficult to see how any researcher could sensibly reach a conclusion about the population prevalence of 'depression'.

In addition to the problem of applying thresholds, there is the question whether to consider the context in which a 'symptom' is reported. There could be a non-disease explanation for whatever is observed, whether the disorder is physical or mental. A skin rash might have been caused by using a certain brand of cosmetic. Loss of appetite might be observed in someone on prison rations. Sleeping too little could be related to drinking too much coffee. The problem is acknowledged in *DSM-5* where it instructs the diagnostician to disregard 'normal sadness or grief'. In effect, it admits that normal circumstances may 'resemble a depressive episode'. As the manual states: 'This decision inevitably requires the exercise of clinical judgement based on the individual's history and the cultural norms for the expression of distress in the context of loss' (2013: 161).

A manual is designed to produce consistency in the diagnostic process, but clinical judgement cannot be checked in routine circumstances. In fact, there is an entirely unacceptable degree of uncertainty about the validity of diagnosis in ordinary settings. As psychiatrist Joel Paris states: 'Major depression is seriously overdiagnosed' (Paris, 2015: 67). The problem has at least been recognised, and according to Horwitz and Wakefield (2007: 6), it *is* possible to distinguish the phenomenon of 'normal sadness' from 'depressive disorder'. They reserve the latter for devastating, profound, and immobilizing suffering that is 'disengaged from actual life circumstances' (ibid.: 12). In their view, this state can persist independently of a context of stress, take on a life of its own, and can be immune to a change in external circumstances (ibid.: 14). Therefore, these authors reserve the concept of 'depressive illness' for a departure from 'biologically designed functionality'.

There is no doubt that depression of a profound degree and of the kind Horwitz and Wakefield describe is not uncommonly seen in psychiatric practice but the

DSM-5 criteria are applied to much milder presentations. Furthermore, the association of profound depression with a biologically disordered mechanism has not yet been established. Horwitz and Wakefield suggest refinements to APA criteria but, in the end, these amount to a diagnostic quibble because they go on to argue that a 'depressive disorder' can arise in the absence of 'any malfunctions in the underlying physiological machinery' (ibid.: 19). If this is so, a disease concept of depression is immune to disproof. Their argument falls apart even further when they suggest that intense normal sadness could always be included under another mental disorder so that suffering patients are still able to take advantage of their health insurance cover (ibid.: 22–23).

The continuum view of depressed mood

One alternative to having an official body stipulate criteria for psychiatric disorders is to administer a questionnaire consisting of a collection of commonly observed forms of distress. Patterns of response can then be identified through statistical analysis of data collected from large representative samples of the population. A depression pattern, partly related to a cluster of anxiety complaints, has been found repeatedly by this technique (e.g. Derogatis, 1975; Crawford and Henry, 2003). However, this method does not provide evidence of depression as a disease entity. The questionnaire items are expressed in ordinary language and consist of phrases such as 'I am disappointed in myself' or 'I feel quite guilty most of the time.' A cluster of so-called symptoms identified statistically could simply reflect a common folk description of distress. Despite this, medical epidemiologists frequently use questionnaires (and also standardised rating scales administered by an interviewer) to survey the incidence and prevalence of 'depressive illness'. If diagnosis of an illness requires clinical judgement, it is not something that can be inferred from self-report or incorporated into rating scales administered by relatively unskilled interviewers. The problem of over- or under-inclusion also exists when the diagnosis is performed by general physicians not trained in psychiatry (Silverstone, 1994; Mojtabai, 2013).

The checklists and scales that have been developed by researchers for different problem areas have their practical uses, especially as a quick way to provide an assessment of key difficulties. Standardised scales can be assessed for their reliability much more conveniently than is the case for diagnoses that rely on clinical judgement. However, reliability is not validity, and the data the scales supply are descriptive. Scores on rating scales have no bearing on whether or not the problems should be conceptualised as illnesses.

In practice, psychometric scales are given more credence than they deserve and end up as indices of 'mental illness'. In their review of the association between social relationships and 'depression', Santini and colleagues (2015) repeat the mantra of the global burden of disease but almost all of the studies they include have employed self-report methods. It is hardly surprising that woefulness is associated with a person's social support, networks, and connectedness. The assumption that this will tell us something about the causes of a disease entity is implausible.

Manuals for psychometric scales suggest cut-off scores that draw a boundary between health and sickness. If 'mental health' were to be defined statistically in this manner, it is impossible to say how many continuous dimensions would be needed to make it up. The scales in common use are usually designed to mirror psychiatric criteria, and so the assumption that they do, in fact, measure 'disorders' is easily made.

The continuum view supposes that there is a spectrum of hedonic states of which depressed mood lies at the negative end and elation (or mania) at the positive end. It is possible that similar causal processes could account for depression and elation at all points along the continuum (Wood, Taylor, and Joseph, 2010). In other words, that 'at the core, they are the same concepts' (Joseph and Wood, 2010: 833). There are three main ways of understanding pathology in relation to a continuum. First, that any example of depressed/elated mood is an expression of a pathological process. This view lacks credibility because depressed mood is so common, people spontaneously recover from it, and analogous behaviour is observed in other animal species. Second, that no state along the continuum need introduce the concept of pathology. Third, that the extreme states can be explained by pathology in a way that does not apply to the middle range. If a disease hypothesis carries any weight, this third position is the most credible.

A different way of looking at how people describe their mood is to view it as a linguistic phenomenon. In other words, very different causal processes may exist across the continuum to produce states that are communicated with a common set of linguistic terms. Experiences may be classified as depressed or elated mood because they share qualities in common even though they have very different causes. There are more than fifteen English words in Roget's thesaurus that describe depressed mood and its antonyms. This suggests that nuances of meaning are not captured by simple scales.

Joseph and Wood (2010: 836) suggest that pathology could be conceptualised in psychological terms but they are reluctant to go the whole way in rejecting the medical model because they cite evidence that low personal well-being is predictive of 'clinical depression' ten years later (Wood and Joseph, 2010). If clinical depression is something that differs from 'very low personal well-being', their continuum view corresponds to the third option set out above.

Joseph and Wood (2010: 837) do call for 'more behaviourally based methods' for assessing negative and positive functioning, and this exposes a problem with the continuum model. The words 'depression' and 'elation' are not clearly linked to behaviour. As commonly used, they do not seem designed to describe a complex behavioural state. For instance, they do not refer explicitly to single features of behaviour such as slow or rapid speech, which is one possible behavioural constituent of depression/elation. Rapidity of speech can vary independently as a personality characteristic seemingly unrelated to mood. In order to produce an adequate description of depressed mood, it would be necessary to include various behavioural components and their situational determinants. Moreover, it is likely that there would be variation across time as well as situations. A person might seem animated or lethargic, smiling or grim-faced, at different moments. Depressed and elated mood might co-exist or alternate; in fact, a cycling mood state is one condition that has been labelled as pathological.

Self-report scales of mood therefore fall short as an adequate depiction of a complex behavioural state. Another criticism of the use of questionnaires is that how a person chooses to present him/herself might reflect their selective employment of language, governed by factors that are not easy to assess (see Chapter 7). Psychiatric criteria for 'depressive disorders' cover a broad range of experiences and behaviour that extend far beyond the way mood is described in everyday situations. Self-report measures endeavour to cover the many signs of the 'illness' of depression but whether they succeed in capturing the psychiatric concept of depression is unclear. Self-reports of mood can be more fairly described as appraisals of how people see themselves as faring in general in a variety of different ways. A continuum of common indicators of mood does not sit easily with the concept of a disease that has the nature of a syndrome.

In their research, Wood, Taylor and Joseph (2010) employed the Center for Epidemiological Studies Depression Scale (CES-D), which is a questionnaire that contains (in addition to depression items) some items that ask about happiness, hope, and enjoyment (Tennant et al., 2007). If a person responds negatively to the positive items, it counts towards their depression score. From their statistical analyses of the correlations between individual items, Wood and colleagues (2010) conclude that there is indeed a continuum from depressed to happy mood rather than two distinct clusters of happy/unhappy states of mind. However, as already noted, continua of linguistic meaning are not descriptions of behaviour, and we cannot be sure that different people are referring to the same thing when they employ semantically related words. If a person is asked how they felt over the previous week, it seems reasonable to suppose that they might have felt happy with some things and depressed about others. It is a gloss on different facets of life. A huge amount of research has been conducted using scales devised on similar lines to the CES-D. Their value as measures of pathology depends on whether variability over the normal range has any implications for theorising about the extremes.

The psychiatric construct of depression is intended to be unitary in the sense that it applies to the state of the whole person over an extended period of time. However, when a person is assessed, the construct quickly breaks down into a number of separate components which are gradually revealed by a detailed inquiry into a person's current circumstances, their biography, physical health, opportunities and constraints on action, life dilemmas, and feedback loops between their acts and their environmental consequences. This raises doubts about the validity of clinical depression as a unitary phenomenon or even a loose syndrome. To abandon a unitary concept of depressive pathology would imply having to raise the game when assessing what 'being depressed' actually means.

Depression/elation as pathology

'Psychotic depression' and 'bi-polar disorder'

The possibility of distinguishing some very severe forms of depressed mood goes back to the beginnings of psychiatry. One of these diagnoses was melancholia, which was amalgamated by Emil Kraepelin with what is now called bi-polar depression (Harris et al., 2011). Other related and severe forms of depressed mood have been called psychotic or endogenous depression. Bi-polar disorder, originally called manic-depression, is currently regarded as a distinct disorder by psychiatrists. It includes those people who have episodes of mania in addition to depressed mood. Although mania is fairly easy to recognise in its extreme form (such as over-activity and pressure of speech), there has been a progressive loosening of diagnostic criteria so that it is now applied to people with milder forms of mania (hypomania), or with rapid changes of mood and emotion that probably have entirely different causes, and to children with behavioural problems (Paris, 2015: 81). Bi-polarity seems to exist on a continuum; the proposal to call it a disease is best limited to those people in whom its main features are incontrovertible.

Although melancholia was eventually merged with MDD, there have been arguments for its reinstatement as a distinct phenotype (Harris et al.: 46). Paris (2015: 75), who is highly sceptical of the MDD diagnosis, is in favour of retaining a diagnosis for severe depression or 'melancholia'. The reality of 'melancholia' is supported by research adopting rigorous criteria for severity and by investigating the life course of people who are admitted to psychiatric institutions where detailed records are kept. It is unlikely that many people will be missed if their depressed mood is sufficiently severe to render them incapable of everyday functioning. Harris and colleagues (2011) managed to work out the incidence of melancholia, diagnosed retrospectively according to ICD10 criteria, in patients who were compulsorily admitted to an asylum in North West Wales in the years 1875–1924. These data were compared with a sample of people from the same area, similarly diagnosed, who used psychiatric services between 1995 and 2005. The recorded information was rich and it was possible to detect prior and future admissions, as well as eventual outcome. Some of the melancholic individuals expressed, in addition, delusional beliefs or hallucinations (i.e. so-called psychotic features).

As might be expected, the incidence of severe depression (all types) in contemporary inpatients was about one-third the rate of mild or moderate depression. The estimated incidence for the melancholic cases who were actually admitted to an institution was less than 1/10,000/year compared with a population incidence for all diagnosed depression of approximately 300–700/10,000/year. In the historical sample, the incidence of inpatients with melancholia was slightly higher than for the contemporary sample. According to historical hospital records, the onset was abrupt with no obvious precipitants, and for almost half the patients the problem had resolved in less than six months; two-thirds had recovered within a year. Followed up (and also traced back) by means of records for ten years, 56 per cent had 'recovered', 6 per cent were still in care, and 30 per cent had died. Remarkably, 87 per cent had

had only one admission over the ten years. In the contemporary sample, hospital stays were very much shorter and the outcome was poorer; over a ten-year period, 58 per cent had been admitted more than once to a psychiatric facility.

It is not unreasonable to describe melancholia as an illness, especially as in the historical sample there was often no clear contextual precipitant for it. However, it is not yet an illness that has been explained by a disease process. As Harris and co-authors note, if episodes of melancholia described in the historical sample 'last several months but commonly resolve within 6–9 months whether treated or not, then suggestions regarding the pathophysiology of melancholic disorders need to incorporate a mechanism that leads to recovery' (2011: 50). It is clearly not enough to lay the blame on inborn errors of metabolism, or indeed on any genetic predisposition as a main cause, that does not also account for the fact that any supposed disease mechanism can be self-correcting. If 84 per cent of the historical sample had only one admission and most recovered within a year without the benefit of electro-convulsive therapy or medication, this does not offer much support for a disease concept or provide a strong case for aggressive physical treatments. On the contrary, it suggests that changes in life circumstances may play an important role in recovery.

Biomarkers of 'pathology'

The assumption that so-called depressive illness has a distinct neuropathology has led to a search for the signs or biomarkers of an underlying disease process (signs of which the person him or herself is normally unaware). The strategy is modelled on medical practice in which a differential diagnosis is based on clinical signs pointing to different pathologies. The search for biomarkers can only be successful if the symptom patterns described in psychiatric diagnostic manuals are in fact the product of discrete sets of biomedical causes. For instance, groups of depressed people are studied as if they are all suffering from the same thing. In a symptomatic sense they are, but a physician would be unlikely to assume that all patients complaining of stomach-ache were suffering from the same disorder. There are likely to be just as many different causes of a complaint of depressed mood. Consequently, any sample of depressed people used in a research study may or may not share similar biomedical signs.

Announcements about the promise of biomedical science have the flavour of a millenarian movement: 'The possibility of harnessing genetic science to head off major depressive disorder, the world's leading cause of disability, is getting closer' (Wilde, 2013). The announcement is then hedged around with provisos. Reports of recent 'promising research' (see below) lament the heterogeneity of the phenomenon they are studying and point to a need to distinguish 'sub-groups'. The hope engendered by an analysis of the human genome that the causes of so-called mental illness will soon be discovered ignores the hugely complex nature of human development (Greenberg, 2011).

Research has been conducted into the sensitivity and specificity of various somatic indicators in groups diagnosed as either depressed or non-depressed (Smith,

Renshaw, and Bilello, 2013). These authors accept that an interview guided by a standardised protocol does not necessarily produce the same diagnostic outcome as one based on clinical judgement. They call for methods to produce an 'accurate' diagnosis (ibid.: 1). However, until such time as criteria are available to identify, reliably and validly, a group (or subgroups) of people complaining of 'depression', there is no means of showing that a new somatic indicator is a valid biomarker of disease.

A recent review article entitled 'The neuroscience of depression' illustrates some of the conceptual difficulties that a brain-based strategy encounters (Singh and Gotlib, 2014). This review was able to reference 177 articles of relatively recent publication, many of which were related to research on the mechanisms of antidepressant medication or other types of physical intervention on the brain. The authors are quick to point out that depression is a heterogeneous disorder and that its measurement is unreliable. As already noted, these limitations must cripple the interpretation of any comparison between groups of 'normal' and 'depressed' individuals. Singh and Gotlib believe that the investigation of 'symptoms' or 'subtypes' of depression may improve matters (ibid.: 69).

The lack of attention to the exact nature of depressive phenomena is in sharp contrast to the precision and sophistication of the measures of brain structure and function adopted in all of the research they review. Despite the smoke and mirrors nature of depression, they continue to assume that the disorder has its own 'pathophysiology' (ibid.: 61). They also refer to 'the depressed brain' (ibid.: 68) and 'the neural benefits of psychotherapy' (ibid.: 67). On their account, the nature of depressed mood will be solved by increasingly precise methods of investigation, but this produces a picture of the world that is analogous to looking through the wrong end of a telescope. We are being led to the absurd conclusion that it will eventually be possible to diagnose depression without having to inquire about the feelings, thoughts, or actions of the sufferer.

The validity of research into neural abnormalities rests on the assumption that it is possible to define a normal (and therefore an abnormal) brain. The authors refer to anomalies while failing to make clear the grounds for establishing normal functions. The concept of a normal brain presumably refers to the brain of a 'normal' person, but in this case normality is a social construct. One alternative would appear to lie in a concept of ideal biological fitness that does not reference social criteria. In practice, much of the data they produce about neural functions is interpreted in terms of general psychological theory that does not reference neural processes.

Some of the evidence these authors review points to 'aberrations in regional brain activation in MDD in response to a variety of emotional and cognitive stimuli, suggesting that depression is associated with dysfunction in emotion regulation' (ibid.: 62). Unless ideal emotion regulation can be specified in biological terms, the findings reflect the way that depressed individuals view the world, something that may show up in brain processes in a rather uninteresting way. In a concluding paragraph, the authors call for innovative examinations of MDD 'that integrate structural and functional properties of the brain in order to provide a strong empirical basis for the development of effective early and lasting interventions that prevent progression and recurrence of MDD' (ibid.: 73). If these interventions involve physical interventions on the brain at an early age before an individual actually demonstrates their 'pathology', the future they envisage is Orwellian. Prevention of 'disease' in this manner seems to carry enormous ethical risks.

Although evidence for a disease model of 'clinical depression' is weak at present, this in no way undermines the potential value of biological research. This research has often been motivated by a search for physical remedies (i.e. it is an offshoot of medicalisation) but this need not be the case. In practice, it is not too difficult to detect biological differences between groups of 'normals' and 'depressed patients'. Lopresti and colleagues (2014) review the evidence on neurotransmitter imbalances, disturbance of the hypothalamic–pituitary–adrenal (HPA) axis, oxidative and nitrosative stress, neuroprogression, mitochondrial disturbances, and immuno-inflammation. All of these areas of investigation are important in their own right, but tying them to a psychiatric diagnosis may simply confuse an interpretation of the findings. I will consider just one example, that of immuno-inflammation.

Research on inflammation of the brain has generated so much interest that a recent review was able to cite around 150 articles (Haapakoski et al., 2016). The body's immune response can be triggered by exposure to bacteria or viruses, but it is also associated with psychological or physiological stress reactions, vigorous exercise, inflammation, trauma, or tissue injury. The authors document complex interactions with the endocrine system and the peripheral and central nervous systems. Interest has been stimulated because 'Preclinical and clinical evidence shows both activation and suppression of immune responses in depressed patients' (ibid.: 67). This evidence is consistent with many hypotheses about the causes or consequences of depressed mood but of key interest is the fact that neuroinflammation occurs after persistent exposure to stressors, with various deleterious effects on neural function. Stressors may, of course, be psychosocial in nature.

In the backstory to the research that Haapakoski and colleagues review is the assumption that 'depression' has its own 'neuropathology'. Inconsistencies or lack of support for hypotheses guiding this research are then explained by the idea that there are different subgroups of depression with their own characteristic neuropathologies. As the authors admit:

> . . . many people with elevated circulating inflammatory markers and/or cortisol levels do not develop depression, suggesting that other factor(s) including stressful life events, childhood trauma, genetic predisposition, comorbid chronic diseases or lifestyle factors may play an important role in the development of depressive symptoms.
>
> *Haapakoski et al., 2016: 69*

It seems likely that a plethora of potential causal factors are implicated but if so, we can ask why an ill-defined psychiatric condition is seen as a useful starting point for research. One motivation in this quest is that of 'identifying sub-groups of depressed patients with increased inflammatory-induced symptoms, who could benefit from immunomodulatory anti-depressive therapies' (ibid.: 68). While hinting at the prospect of new therapies, the authors insert a note of caution when they point out that some of the physiological effects could be a consequence rather than a cause of 'depression'. This is reminiscent of Robert Burton's doubts in 1621 about the direction of causality in the relationship between melancholy and black bile.

Genetic predisposition

A person's genetic inheritance influences just about everything that a person does or experiences and so it would be of little surprise to find some evidence for a genetic predisposition to such a widely recognised phenomenon as depressed mood. According to Lohoff 'twin studies suggest a heritability of 40% to 50%, and family studies indicate a twofold to threefold increase in lifetime risk of developing MDD among first degree relatives' (2010: 539). This does not imply that any single gene has been shown to be necessary or sufficient for MDD. Susceptibility is usually attributed to whole sets of genes, which are probably implicated in other patterns of behaviour as well, both adaptive and maladaptive. Lohoff's review concludes with the remark that the field of psychiatric genetics has been disappointing, with many promising results that fail to be replicated.

With advances in genomics, it is now possible to genotype up to a million SNPs (single nucleotide polymorphisms), which are the most common type of genetic variation among people. In one genome-wide study of depressed versus non-depressed individuals, it was concluded that 'only a large sample comprising more than 50,000 subjects may be sufficiently powered to detect genes for depressive symptoms' (Hek et al., 2013: 667). This study employed the CES-D scale mentioned earlier. One possible explanation for the negative result is the fact that a CES-D score is not a sufficiently precise description of behaviour to show up genetic links because it taps into so many different areas. It may also be susceptible to a variety of influences on self-presentation that have little to do with the construct the scale purports to measure.

The total CES-D score is computed from a number of individual items. The scale is employed in epidemiological surveys and is closely modelled on a *DSM* diagnosis of major depression. The grand total includes items measuring sadness, loss of interest, appetite, sleep, thinking/concentration, guilt, tiredness (fatigue), movement (agitation), and suicidal ideas. The causes of all these aspects of behaviour (assuming that they can be validly measured by self-report) may be sufficiently diverse to render a grand total meaningless from a biological point of view. As we have seen, Fried and Nesse (2015) found that applying the *DSM-5* criteria for MDD yields a very large number of symptom profiles of which 83.9 per cent were endorsed by five or fewer people. They also found that the heterogeneity of profiles was not reduced by taking into account the severity of a person's depressed mood.

A similar negative result regarding a genetic contribution to 'depression' was reached by Ripke and colleagues (2013). However, the Cross-Disorder Group of the Psychiatric Genomics Consortium (CGPGC, 2013) did report SNPs that were associated with psychiatric disorders in genome-wide studies and also similar genetic profiles across some 'disorders'.

One explanation for a failure to find genes for 'depression' is offered by Miller and Yee (2015). They assume, like Kendler (2005), that 'psychopathology' is polygenic. This means that there are a very large number of individual genes that increase risk in a small way, and that only sometimes do 'they converge to make a substantial difference in individual cases' (Miller and Yee, 2015: 264). Put differently, 'a set of rare causal factors or indicators that are uncorrelated in the general population may have a huge impact in the rare cases in which they converge' (ibid.). If this argument holds, the individual cases are unlikely to be reliably detected by such widely used self-report questionnaires as the CES-D or the Hospital Anxiety and Depression Scale (HAD) (Zygmond and Snaith, 1980). The rare 'genetic' cases could be individuals suffering from 'clinical depression' at the severe end of the continuum, but this is not certain. The argument that these individuals are relatively rare provides no support whatsoever for the claim that a large segment of the population is 'mentally ill'.

The authors of a recent review of genetic research into psychiatric disorders conclude that 'the data support multiple novel biological hypotheses' (Sullivan, Daly, and O'Donovan, 2012: 546). This may be so but a biological hypothesis need not relate to disorders or diseases. Nobel Prize winners may show distinct genetic characteristics but they are not, by most accounts, disordered. Sullivan and colleagues (2012) are convinced that psychiatric disorders are fundamentally diseases; a more realistic view is that they are ways of describing phenotypes – that is, the observable expression of an interaction between genetic make-up and environment. A genetic disease is assumed to result from an abnormality in an individual's genome, a rather rare occurrence. Genes may predispose a person to develop a disease, probably in conjunction with particular environmental influences; however, a predisposition is not a disorder. Whatever is revealed by future research is likely to be a complex interaction between biology and an adverse environment.

Psychosocial correlates of depressed mood

There is strong evidence that a person's depressed mood is related to external circumstances and life adversities. It is known that women are twice as likely as men to receive a diagnosis of depression. This higher prevalence could be related to experiences associated with the female role, but attempts have been made to explain it biologically (see below). In general, the greater the association of depressed mood with psychosocial variables, the less credible is a disease explanation.

According to one view, it has been assumed that certain behaviour patterns that underlie depressed mood have been selected as biologically advantageous over the course of human evolution. It is additionally assumed that these evolved traits could give rise to problems in contemporary societies when they no longer fulfil a functional role and have maladaptive consequences (Durisko, Mulsant, and Andrews, 2015; Nesse and Ellsworth, 2009). In archaic environments, 'depressive-type behaviour' may have been adaptive by serving to avoid risk, conserve energy, minimise losses, and reallocate resources to the analysis of situations in which an individual's goals are blocked. Another behaviour pattern widely observed in animal species that have dominance hierarchies is 'giving in' (i.e. conceding social defeat) and soliciting resources from others (e.g. begging, crying, agitation, self-harm, and helplessness). Durisko and colleagues (2015) interpret all these evolved traits as pathways to the development of 'depressive disorders', although it is not clear why their expression should be viewed as pathology. Presumably, a behaviour pattern persists longer than is necessary or becomes overgeneralised, in which case the 'pathology' probably lies in maladaptive learning processes, involving vicious cycle feedback loops. Theorists who adopt an evolutionary perspective rarely refer to the evolution of general systems of communication that enable humans to relate discriminations of, say, social rank, to completely unrelated situations, such as objects on a chessboard or dolls in a toy cupboard. The source of maladjustment could, with equal justification, be attributed to the maladaptive use of arbitrary signs.

Epidemiological research

The methods employed by epidemiologists take it as given that the main task is to study the incidence and prevalence of diseases, and their search for causes includes psychosocial variables. In psychiatric epidemiology, it is assumed that disorders are analogous to diseases.

In a paper entitled 'Size and burden of depressive disorders in Europe', Paykel and colleagues acknowledge some of the methodological problems of assessment and definition (Paykel, Brugha, and Fryers, 2005). They state that the term depression 'covers a spectrum ranging from a normal mood of unhappiness to an abnormal, severe and incapacitating disorder' (ibid.: 411). It is argued that there are no clear-cut demarcation points along the continuum. Paykel and colleagues are also uncertain that there is a single continuum. They refer to a possibly distinct, mild and mixed 'disorder' that includes 'anxiety symptoms'.

Despite their methodological concerns, they confidently provide evidence about the prevalence of 'major depression' in different European countries. The data point to a figure of between 1.8 per cent and 9 per cent of the adult population. Women consistently show higher rates than men in a ratio of around 2:1. People who are afflicted in this manner are called 'depressives', as if this was a clearly delineated section of the population. The authors finally announce that 'depression produces substantial economic costs' (ibid.: 415). They believe that 'major advances are likely in the next 20 years in knowledge of aetiology of depression' (ibid.: 417), and, in this connection, they mention genetic studies and brain-scanning techniques.

The authors do not expect similar advances in changing the psychosocial correlates of 'depression', although these are evident in the statistics. Aside from the gender ratio already mentioned, other associations with prevalence are age (rising from adolescence, peaking in middle age and then reducing), urban living, stressful life events, lack of social support, a less privileged social position, low material resources, less education, and unemployment. A diagnosis of depression is also associated with physical illness and with the diagnosis of other mental illnesses. In their résumé, the authors state that:

> The best established social causes, such as life events and poor social support, seem in many cases inevitable consequences of the life cycle, or of family relationships, particularly in affluent and settled circumstances, but less so in groups and areas under marked social adversity.
>
> *Paykel et al., 2005: 418*

It would seem more reasonable to assume that these social causes are at least potentially more modifiable and less inevitable than the genetic causes or brain dysfunctions the authors confidently expect to be discovered.

In another review of 'the increasing burden of depression', Lépine and Briley (2011) examine evidence on recurrence of the problem, the economic burden, and the significantly increased mortality risk, especially for suicide, which is 20–27 times higher than in the general population. They conclude that 'as the infectious diseases, especially in developing countries, are progressively controlled, depression is predicted to become the major health burden worldwide' (ibid.: 6). They also note that up to 50 per cent of severe cases in developed countries, and up to 85 per cent in less-developed counties, receive no treatment (ibid.: 3). It is probably no coincidence that one of the authors is a director of NeuroBiz Consulting and Communication, and describes himself on its website as having had 24 years' experience in the pharmaceutical industry, with particular expertise in the area of research, development, and marketing of antidepressants. We are reminded of Robert Burton's caution about 'quack empirics'. As Paris remarks: 'The unitary theory [of MDD] also had a hidden agenda, in that it implied that patients with major depression should receive the same treatment, that is, antidepressants. It provided an ideological basis for prescribing drugs to people who are unhappy' (2015: 69).

A study of the incidence of depression recorded in primary care settings in the UK found that *diagnoses* decreased between the years 1996–2006 while recorded *complaints* of depressed mood increased (Rait et al., 2009). This suggests that general practitioners have become less inclined to diagnose rather than simply record complaints. The combined figures remained fairly constant at 24.8/1000 person-years at risk (PYAR), equivalent to a mean annual incidence of 2.5 per cent. Judging by rising levels of prescription of antidepressants (HSCIC, 2015), this has little to do with diagnosis of a disease but is simply a quick way of dealing with a large number of people for whom alternative forms of intervention are unavailable.

Psychosocial 'risk factors'

The medical perspective on depression as an illness is that certain psychosocial events, adversities, or personality characteristics could raise the risk of contracting the illness. In the case of physical disease, it is assumed that epidemiological studies may help to reveal pathological causes and point towards sensible preventative measures. We now know that it is inadvisable to drink water conducted in lead pipes or to smoke cigarettes. A causal pathway between these practices and a known effect on the body can be traced. A medical risk factor can, of course, be defined without it necessarily leading to negative consequences (e.g. smoking cigarettes).

A similar rationale for studying the antecedents of so-called mental illnesses is less convincing because the end-points are extremely varied patterns of behaviour which have few obvious empirical links to causal processes. In other words, to discover provoking events and vulnerabilities for becoming depressed may tell us little or nothing about depression as a so-called pathology. The chief analytical problem is that of dissecting out personal, social, and biological influences in what must be a complex and dynamic system. I will take one set of studies to illustrate a general argument about the methodological problems. In landmark research on depression amongst women in an inner London borough, Brown and Harris (1978) found an association between depressed mood and four vulnerability factors, namely having three or more children under the age of 14 at home, absence of an intimate confiding relationship, lack of employment outside the home, and the loss of a mother before age 11. Brown and Harris found that depressed mood was much more likely to follow an adverse life event in vulnerable rather than in non-vulnerable women. The adverse event could be seen as equivalent in medical terms to a pathogen provoking disease.

The results of this study have not been consistently replicated. Patten (1991) aggregated the findings of four very similar studies with the Brown and Harris data and concluded that all four vulnerability factors raise the odds of experiencing depressed mood, even when the effect of provoking events is disregarded. The odds for developing depressed mood were raised by between 1.7 and 2.0 for the Brown and Harris factors. This suggests that a provoking event is not analogous to, say, a pathogen causing illness. It is just one more element in the mix. Patten's analysis examined each vulnerability separately and this type of analysis does not consider their combined effect, which could be multiplicative rather than additive. The 'mix' for any so-called mental illness may be crucial. Put differently, the patterning of reciprocal causal interactions, including their temporal sequencing, could be crucial in the individual case. A depressed mood is not really an 'end-point' like an illness, because its influence reverberates throughout other causal influences. Researchers are now attempting to conceptualise complex interactions with network models (Borsboom and Cramer, 2013). The underlying concept is that of a dynamic system, not linear causality.

The number of variables that can be included in an epidemiological survey is bound to be limited and some might be excluded because the researcher has not envisaged their importance. Vulnerabilities for depressed mood may also be 'risk factors' for many other so-called disorders, which are not recorded if not looked for.

Brown and Harris went to great efforts, through careful analysis of their qualitative interviews, to establish meaningful descriptors for their observations. However, the absence of vulnerability factors could be interpreted as sources of strengths that foster an upbeat mood. Having a caring partner, being able to meet the demands of a smaller number of children (and therefore enjoy them more), and having ongoing support from a mother figure could all be viewed as positive assets. It is open to interpretation whether the loss of a mother before age 11 has cascading negative effects leading to depressed mood, or whether the presence of a mother who is able to share the care of children lifts the burden and stress of parenthood (both effects are of course possible). Taking Brown and Harris's four vulnerabilities, a good novelist could construct a very large number of life stories out of them. We might want to question whether or not a woman chose to have three or more children. Were they the product of a supportive partnership that failed, or did a woman choose to have children in the absence of a supportive partner? Was the lack of an intimate partner related to a woman's preferences and/or the result of earlier bad experiences with men? To what extent does a woman's depressed mood bring about consequences such as a disinterest in social activities that further consolidates her vulnerability?

Numerical methods in epidemiology are based on group data (rather than the circumstances of unique individuals identified as ill) and it is assumed that 'mental illness', as a biomedical event, can be predicted from mathematical equations that quantify variables such as age, social class, parenting, and adverse developmental events. The statistical computations can examine the influence of one variable while controlling for another, and also show how two or more variables interact. However, from this aggregated group data, it is not known how the variables play out in the life of a single individual. At an individual level of analysis, how A interacts with B given C is a dynamic interaction that is best investigated by conducting a qualitative interview. Of course, it is reasonable to expect that a unique personal trajectory would broadly conform to a general pattern. However, the idiographic approach to research differs from the nomothetic in the kind of reasoning it employs. Sarbin, Taft and Bailey (1960: 256) point out differences between qualitative analysis and statistical prediction based on a set of variables in grouped data. The centrality of a concept of self in Jahoda's (1958) review of ideas about psychological health (see Chapter 7) is a reminder of the importance of the idiographic (person) level of analysis. Valuable as general etiological models are, investigators would have little idea what to include as predictor variables in their equations unless they had gleaned them from an intimate and direct acquaintance with the past and present lives of individuals in a state of woe. Ideally, a means of modelling the interaction of variables at the person-level is needed in addition to interactions at the group level (Hallam, 2013).

These reservations about the interpretation of numerical data suggest that qualitative life history research might be more informative. It may be possible to draw out general themes that characterise a particular kind of problem. Observations can be refined until something like a theoretical model is developed (e.g. by using a method such as grounded theory – Birks and Mills, 2015). Whatever that model turns out to be, it is unlikely to resemble a model of the causes of a physical disease. The end-state is not a discrete illness, and so linking it to presuppositions about risks and vulnerabilities is doubly difficult. The process of discovery in medicine is more likely to point to a trail of mediating events and processes that link antecedent causes to somatic pathology (e.g. what a particular microorganism does to the body). In the case of a demonstrable connection between, say, childhood physical or sexual abuse and later psychological problems, we are still left in the dark about the causal links. The existence of associations between childhood adversities and later woes is a valuable starting point but when choosing how to investigate them, a template taken from medicine may have limited value (van den Hout, 2014).

There is no shortage of evidence to associate developmental events with later woes. Maniglio, in his review of studies that trace the long-term effects of child sexual abuse (CSA) on 'anxiety disorders', describes what he is doing as developing a 'multifactorial etiological model' (2012: 96). He concludes that CSA is a risk factor, and equally so for males and females. He also observes that it may not be related to the severity of abuse, and that other variables may interact or act independently to cause 'anxiety disorders'. Clearly, reviews of this kind of research have implications for primary prevention. However, Maniglio recommends that future research should examine how different variables interact over time, and how abuse survivors manage to overcome their adversities and compensate for them. A qualitative approach seems best suited for this purpose.

With regard to 'depression', Colman and colleagues (2014) drew conclusions from surveys that followed a group of children into adulthood from 1946 to 1999. The researchers found that childhood deprivation and stressors had important direct and indirect effects on later 'depression'. As with CSA, further insight into the complexity of the developmental process is needed.

With regard to public policies aimed at prevention, the most important adversities and vulnerabilities are ones that have a high probability of interacting with provoking events to cause significant distress, problems, or illness. If it is possible to influence the crucial predictors, investment in primary prevention might be worthwhile when the benefits outweigh the costs. However, if as seems likely, there are a large number of potentially relevant and interacting variables, unique outcomes may be difficult to predict. For instance, a vulnerability such as extreme shyness or impulsivity might not manifest itself later on as distress or problematic conduct, depending on other circumstances. A person's 'Achilles heel' is not necessarily revealed if she or he is fortunate enough not to encounter a critical provoking event (e.g. a road traffic accident or an abusive partner). In other words, chance or fate must play a large part in many woes.

Pathways to physical illness are complicated enough, but the developmental causes of other woes are even more difficult to tease apart or model mathematically (O'Connor, 2015). Psychological strengths and vulnerabilities could be the causes or consequences of other biological, social, or pathology variables or their interaction. Psychosocial causes could come into play very early on in life but only produce their consequences later in adulthood. Events that have an enduring effect could be expressed either through behavioural or neurophysiological pathways (or both) and then interact with later provocations. A person's genetic inheritance might contribute directly to or, more likely, interact with other factors.

Depression and gender

The large gender imbalance in diagnostic and questionnaire measures of so-called depression calls for explanation. It is worth pointing out that although women are more likely to report depressed mood, men are more likely to carry out an intention to end their own life, especially during downturns in the economic cycle (Reeves, McKee, and Stuckler, 2014). Although there is a higher prevalence of 'depression' amongst women in general population samples and in service users of the mental health system, for healthy men and women who are not in a woeful state, mean depression scores on a well-validated psychometric scale were found to be identical in one study of dizygotic and monozygotic twins (Burton et al., 2015). The overall estimate for a genetic contribution to variance in depression scores was also the same for both sexes.

Freeman and Freeman (2013) have reviewed possible causes of the gender imbalance in the prevalence of so-called depression. These authors seem quite content to muddy any distinction between well-being, mental health, and mental illness. They refer to the General Health Questionnaire (GHQ-12 – Goldberg, 1992), which was designed to detect 'symptoms' of anxiety and depression, as 'a measure of psychological well-being', and they call for 'an assessment that covers all the key areas' in order to give 'an overall picture of mental health' (Freeman and Freeman, 2013: 67). If the distinction between well-being and mental illness is unimportant, there is little point in continuing to use medical terminology, such as diagnosed depression. Moreover, there is a world of difference between calling a woman 'dissatisfied' or 'discontented', and calling her 'disordered'.

Freeman and Freeman (2013: 69) cite evidence to show that women's rated happiness has been declining relative to men since the 1970s, in which period it exceeded men's happiness levels (Stevenson and Wolfers, 2009). If 'unhappiness' can be equated with a diagnosis of 'depression' (MDD), one would expect similar trends across time in relation to the higher odds ratio for female depression relative to men's. That is, the odds ratio should be increasing since the 1970s.

This expectation is inconsistent with the findings from surveys conducted in 15 countries in which the higher odds for MDD among women were less pronounced in more recent age cohorts (Seedat et al., 2009). A measure was obtained for traditional gender roles in each country and it was found that the higher prevalence of MDD in women decreased as female gender roles become less traditional. According to a speculation of the authors:

> In the case of MDD, the gender roles hypothesis would interpret our findings as meaning that increases in female opportunities in the domains of employment, birth control, and other indicators of increasing gender role equality promote improvements in female mental health by reducing exposure to stressors that can lead to depression and by increasing access to effective stress-buffering resources.
>
> *Seedat et al., 2009: 793*

It is expecting a great deal to explain the psychological effects of major changes in gender roles, taking into account education and employment opportunities for women across several generations. Change can mean greater opportunity but also the possibility of greater frustration if change is resisted. In any event, measuring the response to change in terms of the prevalence of psychiatric disorders would seem to be a very blunt research tool, especially when 'mental illness' is confounded with low well-being.

One example of a single adversity of potential significance is childhood sexual abuse. This is more commonly inflicted upon girls than upon boys, and therefore could potentially account for the fact that the rate of so-called depression is higher in adult women. A UK general population survey found that 5.2 per cent of women reported a history of sexual abuse as against 1.6 per cent of men. There is a strong link with later suicide amongst women (Freeman and Freeman, 2013: 121). These authors re-analysed data from a later, 2007, UK Adult Psychiatric Morbidity Survey (NCSR, 2011) to examine the relationship between a history of sexual abuse and the greater odds of women developing 'depression'. Adjusting statistically for a history of abuse, the odds were only reduced from 1.6 to 1.5 (Freeman and Freeman, 2013: 140). Similarly, a number of other adverse events, taken singly, had only a small effect on the odds ratio. One explanation for this finding of the apparent slight effect of abuse is that severe woes may result from multiple adverse circumstances acting together, and quite possibly in a multiplicative way rather than in an additive fashion. This is the position adopted by Hyde, Mezulis, and Abramson (2008) in their review of explanatory models of the gender ratio for 'depression'. These authors disregard any potential difference between continuum and categorical descriptions of 'depression', implying that they reject the existence of pathological depressive sub-groups. Although this may be the correct view to take, there is the risk that the concept of 'depression' can end up meaning almost any form of distress that lowers mood. Their systemic dynamic theoretical model that includes a variety of interacting factors is likely to become more and more complex and end up as a 'theory of everything'.

As there are hormonal differences between men and women, researchers have picked on this as a potential differential risk factor. Antenatal and post-natal depressed mood have been a particular focus for research. In a review of evidence for maternal depression, anxiety, and stress during pregnancy, Biaggi and colleagues (2016) note that this is a period of hormonal change as well as stimulation of the hypothalamic–pituitary–adrenal (HPA) axis and the inflammatory system. Activation of these systems may have long-term effects on the mother and the baby's development (Glover, 2015). The study found that the chief correlates of antenatal depression or anxiety were a previous history of anxiety and depression, childhood parenting experiences, child abuse, lack of social support, young age, low educational achievement, unemployment, ethnicity, adverse life events, and unplanned/unwanted pregnancy. There is nothing in this list that points to depression as a disorder or disease.

As regards, post-partum depression, Halbreich and Karkun (2006) found a high degree of cross-cultural variability, with prevalence rates between 0 per cent and almost 60 per cent. This suggests that its determinants are highly variable as well.

For non-medically oriented researchers, the reasons for depressed mood in women are sought in social factors. Stoppard and McMullin (2003), summarising the contributions to their edited book, point to demoralisation stemming from betrayal by significant figures in a woman's life, a normal response to losses following childbirth, attempts to live up to the cultural roles expected of women and mothers, and difficulty expressing anger through dialogue. As Stoppard and McMullin argue:

> . . . their [women's] resistance to these cultural narratives often took the form of chastising themselves for having fallen victim to these narratives, stating that it was their own responsibility to move beyond them, or seeking forms of treatment or intervention that were focussed on individual change.
>
> *Stoppard and McMullin, 2003: 210*

A woman's accommodation to the demands placed upon her through self-blame is made easier by the availability of diagnoses and a mental health system that makes an illness interpretation of her woes seem appropriate. As these authors go on to say:

> . . . focusing on changing one's self is seen as possible, whereas effecting change in discriminatory attitudes and expectations, violence toward and abuse of women, poverty, and inadequate employment opportunities is viewed either as improbable or as a very difficult and slow process.
>
> *Ibid.*

It's worth noting that self-blame has been interpreted as a symptom of a depressive disorder.

Summary

'Major depression' has been proclaimed to be one of the most disabling diseases in the world, notwithstanding great difficulty in establishing that this so-called disorder is a unitary syndrome of signs and symptoms. A consensus has not yet been achieved on whether depressed/elated mood can be represented along a single continuum or whether it is possible to distinguish categories of mood states that are discontinuous with normal variation. Research into the biological correlates of diagnosed depression is seriously hampered by the aforementioned definitional problems. The prevalence of diagnosed depression is strongly associated with childhood adversity, various indicators of social disadvantage, and the female gender. So far, there is little evidence to show that this higher prevalence is linked to biomedical variables. However, it is a considerable challenge to model the interaction between biological, social, and psychological factors during human development, and so the optimal method for investigating depressed mood still remains an open question.

References

Biaggi, A., Conroy, S., Pawlby, S. & Pariante, C. M. (2016) Identifying the women at risk of antenatal anxiety and depression: A systematic review. *Journal of Affective Disorders*. 191, pp.62–77.

Birks, M. & Mills, J. (2015) *Grounded theory (Practical guide)*. London, Sage.

Borsboom, D. & Cramer, A. O. (2013) Network analysis: An integrative approach to the structure of psychopathology. *Annual Review of Clinical Psychology*. 9, pp.91–121.

Brown, G. W. & Harris, T. O (1978) *Social origins of depression: A study of psychiatric disorder in women*. London, Tavistock Publications.

Burton, K. L., Williams, L. M., Clark, C. et al. (2015) Sex differences in the shared genetics of dimensions of self-reported depression and anxiety. *Journal of Affective Disorders*. 188, pp.35–42.

CGPGC (2013) Cross-Disorder Group of the Psychiatric Genomics Consortium: Genetic relationship between five psychiatric disorders estimated from genome-wide SNPs. *Nature Genetics*. 45(9), pp.984–994.

Colman, I., Jones, P. B., Kuh, D. et al. (2014) Early development, stress and depression across the life course: Pathways to depression in a national British birth cohort. *Psychological Medicine*. 44(13), pp.2845–2854.

Crawford, J. R. & Henry, J. D. (2003) The Depression Anxiety Stress Scales (DASS): Normative data and latent structure in a large non-clinical sample. *British Journal of Clinical Psychology*. 42(2), pp.111–131.

Derogatis, L. R. (1975) *The brief symptom inventory*. Baltimore, MD, Clinical Psychometric Research.

DSM-5 (2013) *Diagnostic and statistical manual of mental disorders (DSM-5)*. Arlington, VA, American Psychiatric Association.

Durisko, Z., Mulsant, B. H. & Andrews, P. W. (2015) An adaptionist perspective on the etiology of depression. *Journal of Affective Disorders*. 172, pp.315–323.

Freeman, D. & Freeman, J. (2013) *The stressed sex: Uncovering the truth about men, women, and mental health*. Oxford, Oxford University Press.

Fried, E. I. (2016) Depression – more than the sum of its symptoms, *The Psychologist*. 29(1), pp.42–43.

Fried, E. I. & Nesse, R. M. (2015) Depression is not a consistent syndrome: An investigation of unique symptom patterns in the STAR*D study. *Journal of Affective Disorders*. 172, pp.96–102.

Glover, V. (2015) Prenatal stress and its effects on the fetus and the child: Possible underlying biological mechanisms. *Advances in Neurobiology*. 10, pp.269–283.

Goldberg, D. (1992) *General health questionnaire (GHQ-12)*. Windsor, UK, NFER-Nelson.

Greenberg, G. (2011) The failure of biogenetic analysis in psychology: Why psychology is not a biological science. *Research in Human Development*. 8, pp.173–191.

Haapakoski, R., Ebmeier, K. P., Alenius, H. & Kivimäki, M. (2016) Innate and adaptive immunity in the development of depression: An update on current knowledge and technological advances. *Progress in Neuro-Psychopharmacology and Biological Psychiatry*. 66, pp.63–72.

Halbreich, U. & Karkun, S. (2006) Cross-cultural and social diversity of prevalence of postpartum depression and depressive symptoms. *Journal of Affective Disorders*. 91, pp.97–111.

Hallam, R. S. (2013) *Individual case formulation*. Oxford, Academic Press.

Harris, M. et al. (2011) The incidence and prevalence of admissions for melancholia in two cohorts (1875–1924 and 1995–2005). *Journal of Affective Disorders*. 134, pp.45–51.

Hek, K., Demirkan, A., Lahti, J. et al. (2013) A genome-wide association study of depressive symptoms. *Biological Psychiatry*. 73(7), pp.667–678.

Horwitz, A. V. & Wakefield, J. C. (2007) *The loss of sadness: How psychiatry transformed normal sorrow into depressive disorder*. New York, Oxford University Press.

HSCIC (2015) *Prescriptions dispensed in the community in England, 2004–2014*. Health and Social Care Information Centre, 7 July. Available from: www.hscic.gov.uk. [Accessed 12 December 2016].

Hyde, J. H., Mezulis, A. H. & Abramson, L. Y. (2008) The ABCs of depression: Integrating affective, biological, and cognitive models to explain the emergence of the gender difference in depression. *Psychological Review*. 115(2), pp.291–313.

Jahoda, M. (1958) *Current concepts of positive mental health*. New York, Basic Books.

Joseph, S. & Wood, A. (2010) Assessment of positive functioning; Theoretical and practical issues. *Clinical Psychology Review*. 30, pp.830–838.

Kendler, K. S. (2005) "A gene for . . . ?: The nature of gene action in psychiatric disorders. *American Journal of Psychiatry*. 162, pp.1243–1252.

Lépine, J.-P. & Briley, M. (2011). The increasing burden of depression. *Neuropsychiatric Disease and Treatment*, 7 (Suppl. 1), pp.3–7.

Lohoff, F. W. (2010) Overview of the genetics of major depressive disorder. *Current Psychiatry Reports*. 12(6), pp.539–546.

Lopresti, A. L., Maker, G. L., Hood, S. D. & Drummond, P. D. (2014) A review of peripheral biomarkers in major depression: The potential of inflammatory and oxidative stress biomarkers. *Progress in Neuropsychopharmacology and Biological Psychiatry*. 48, pp.102–111.

Lynch, T. (2015) *Depression delusion, Volume One: The myth of the brain chemical imbalance*. Limerick, Mental Health Publishing.

Maniglio, R. (2012) Child sexual abuse in the etiology of anxiety disorders: A systematic review of reviews. *Trauma, Violence, and Abuse*. 14(2), pp.96–112.

Mathers, C. D. & Loncar, D. (2006) Projections of global mortality and burden of disease from 2002 to 2030. *PLoS Med*, 3(11), e442.

McMullen, L. M. & Stoppard, J. M. (2003) Conclusion. In: Stoppard, J. M. & McMullen, L. M. (eds.), *Situating sadness: Women and depression in social context*. New York, New York University Press, pp.207–215.

Miller, G. A. & Yee, C. M. (2015) Moving psychopathology forward. *Psychological Inquiry*. 26(3), pp.263–267.

Mojtabai, R. (2013) Clinician-identified depression in community settings: Concordance with structured-interview diagnoses. *Psychotherapy and Psychosomatics*, 82, pp.161–169.

Moore, M., Yuen, H. M., Dunn, N. et al. (2009) Explaining the rise in antidepressant prescribing: A descriptive study using the general practice research database. *British Medical Journal*, 339, b3999.

Moussavi, S. et al. (2007) Depression, chronic diseases, and decrements in health: Results from the World Health Surveys. *The Lancet*. 370(9590), pp.851–858.

NCSR (2011) National Centre for Social Research, *Adult Psychiatric Morbidity Survey, 2007*, 3rd edn. Colchester, Essex: UK Data Archive SN: 6379.

Nesse, R. M. & Ellsworth, P. C. (2009) Evolution, emotions, and emotional disorders. *American Psychologist*. 64, pp.129–139.

O'Connor, K., Robert, M., Pérodeau, G. & Seguin, M. (2015) Trajectory-based methods in clinical psychology: A person centred narrative approach. *New Ideas in Psychology*. 39, pp.12–22.

Paris, J. (2015) *Overdiagnosis in psychiatry: How modern psychiatry lost its way while creating a diagnosis for almost all of life's misfortunes*. Oxford, Oxford University Press.

Patten, S. B. (1991) Are the Brown and Harris "vulnerability factors" risk factors for depression? *Journal of Psychiatry and Neuroscience*. 16(5), pp.267–271.

Paykel, E. S., Brugha, T. & Fryer, T. (2005) Size and burden of depressive disorders in Europe. *European Neuropsychopharmacology*. 15, pp.411–423.

Pilgrim, D. & Bentall, R. (1999) The medicalisation of misery: A critical realist analysis of the concept of depression. *Journal of Mental Health*. 8(3), pp.262–274.

Rait, G. et al. (2009) Recent trends in the incidence of recorded depression in primary care. *British Journal of Psychiatry*. 195(6), pp.520–524.

Reeves, A., McKee, M. & Stuckler, D. (2014) Economic suicides in the great recession in Europe and North America. *British Journal of Psychiatry*. 205(3), pp.246–247.

Ripke, S., Wray, N. R., Lewis, C. M. et al. (2013) A mega-analysis of genome-wide association studies for major depressive disorder. *Molecular Psychiatry*. 18(4), pp.497–511.

Santini, Z. I., Koyanagi, A., Tyrovolas, S. & Mason, C. (2015) The association between social relationships and depression: A systematic review. *Journal of Affective Disorders*. 175, pp.53–65.

Sarbin, T. R., Taft, R. & Bailey, D. E. (1960). *Clinical inference and cognitive theory*. Oxford, Holt, Rinehart, and Winston.

Seedat, S. et al. (2009) Cross-national associations between gender and mental disorders in the World Health Organization World Mental Health Surveys. *Archives of General Psychiatry*. 66, pp.785–795.

Silverstone, P. H. (1994) Poor efficacy of the hospital anxiety and depression scale in the diagnosis of major depressive disorder in both medical and psychiatric patients. *Journal of Psychosomatic Research*. 38(5), pp.441–450.

Singh, M. K. & Gotlib, I. H. (2014) The neuroscience of depression: Implications for assessment and intervention. *Behaviour Research and Therapy*. 62, pp.60–73.

Smith, K. M., Renshaw, P. F. & Bilello, J. (2013) The diagnosis of depression: Current and emerging methods. *Comprehensive Psychiatry*. 54(1), pp.1–6.

Stevenson, B. & Wolfers, J. (2009) The paradox of declining female happiness. *American Economic Journal: Economic Policy, American Economic Association*. 1(2), pp.190–225.

Sullivan, P. F., Daly, M. J. & O'Donovan, M. (2012) Genetic architectures of psychiatric disorders: The emerging picture and its implications. *Nature Reviews: Genetics*. 13(8), pp.537–551.

Tennant, R. et al. (2007) The Warwick-Edinburgh Mental Well-being Scale (WEMWBS): Development and UK validation. *Health and Quality of Life Outcome*. 5, p.63.

van den Hout (2014) Psychiatric symptoms as pathogens. *Clinical Neuropsychiatry*. 11(6), pp.153–159.

WHO (2015) Fact sheet on depression No 369. Available from: www.who.int/mediacentre/factsheets/fs369/en/ [Accessed 10 May 2017].

Wilde, A. (2013) Predicting the risk of depressive disorder – promises and pitfalls. *The Conversation*, 22 January. Available from: https://theconversation.com/predicting-the-risk-of-depressive-disorder-promises-and-pitfalls-1097 [Accessed 10 May 2017].

Wood, A. E. & Joseph, S. (2010) The absence of positive psychological (eudaimonic) well-being as a risk factor for depression: A ten year cohort study. *Journal of Affective Disorders*. 122, pp.213–217.

Wood, A. E., Taylor, P. J. & Joseph, S. (2010) Does the CES-D measure a continuum from depression to happiness? Comparing substantive and artifactual models. *Psychiatry Research*. 177, pp.120–123.

Zygmond, A. S. & Snaith, R. P. (1980) The Hospital Anxiety and Depression Scale, *Acta Psychiatrica Scandinavica*. 67, pp.361–370.

5

AGENCY, RATIONALITY, AND THE CONCEPT OF MENTAL ILLNESS

When Szasz argued that mental illness is a myth, I do not believe that he was suggesting that societies could do without myths. It was to claim that the word 'illness', in the phrase 'mental illness', was a metaphor. The aim of this chapter is to discuss how a belief that another person (or oneself) is mentally ill is related to a belief in 'free will', a belief that seems to incorporate an element of mythology. An ability to exercise choice is fundamental to the definition of all woes. A woe denotes a state of affairs in which a person typically acts, thinks, or feels in ways that are upsetting to self or others. Attempts to redress this state of affairs often turn out to be self-defeating, and the person becomes resigned to bearing a burden of distress. Mental illness is put forward as one explanation for this kind of departure from a state of mind or behaviour that is classed as freely chosen and accords with whatever is considered reasonable or acceptable. In past eras, a person might have believed that their will had been taken over by a superior power, such as a god or demon.

As an assumed ability, 'free will' is mythical in the sense that being in possession of a 'will' that freely chooses is not something that can, at present, be translated into terms that would satisfy a natural scientist. At best, we can trace the development during childhood of a capacity to choose freely and assess this against social criteria marking its accomplishment. Although the way in which 'free will' is acquired may not be transparent, a belief in it (as some kind of human faculty) is something that most people take for granted. In this chapter, I will assume that a belief in 'free will' performs a socially necessary function, and follow Ryle (1949) in asserting that will or volition is an after-the-fact description for a certain class of behaviour that has to be learned in childhood. In other words, it is not an ability with which humans are naturally endowed but a product of how we are socialised. Of course, humans, like all animals, have certain 'natural' agentive powers. At its most basic level, individuals engage in voluntary behaviour when they acquire the capacity to indicate a request, accede to a request, or refuse it. This kind of behaviour is observable in primates and pre-verbal infants. In the failures of agency that are now explained as mental illness, a person cannot easily implement what they want to do or stop doing what they (or others), do not want (them) to do.

After elaborating the role of agency in so-called mental illness, I discuss the special case in which coercion is employed in an attempt to change the way a person behaves in order to protect others or the person him or herself. Coercion, if used at all, is usually confined to what could be termed the 'hard cases' of so-called mental illness, although the great majority of people labelled mentally disordered are, in reality, 'soft cases' – that is, people who recognise the need to make a change but have difficulty in doing so. I discuss how these two groups of people have been labelled, the kinds of explanation that are produced for failures 'to adjust', and criticise attempts to normalise mental illness as just another kind of illness that anyone might happen to suffer from.

Agency and attribution in so-called mental illness

Most people, most of the time, do acquire the ability to adjust their behaviour to bring it in line with their own wishes or to take account of the distress or annoyance it might cause others. If they are unable to do so, the inability may appear, even to them, as surprising and inexplicable. This kind of situation is nothing out of the ordinary. It develops into a state of so-called mental ill-health only when a person fails to find a way of successfully resolving it. A person might then be viewed as lacking resilience or self-determination, or as having a character weakness, such as being oversensitive or easily overwhelmed. In making these social judgements, other people are often ignorant about the impact that a woe is capable of having or what it is that makes a person particularly susceptible to it.

People are often reluctant to attribute their failure to act 'reasonably' to causes outside of their own control. They hold a conviction that their power of volition or their 'free will' should suffice to ensure that they are able to govern themselves rationally, morally, or wisely. Right living – that which promotes the good life and lessens the chance of experiencing woes – is thought to depend on freely exercised 'right choices'. People are held (or hold themselves) accountable when they fail to live up to their own or others' expectations. The State assumes this to be the case and so its methods include incentives for behaving well and disincentives for behaving badly. The Law may be employed to bolster our personal powers, which are prone to slippage. For instance, it requires a law and penalties to ensure use of a seat belt when driving a car. The ability to choose reasonably is not, therefore, simply an internal power because it has to be propped up by a system of social consequences. In the presence of sanctions, we 'freely choose' to attach a seat belt and feel that this is a matter of our own volition, having accepted the rationale for belting up. However, when we disagree with the rationale for a sanction, the latter may be experienced as coercive.

'Hard and soft' cases of so-called mental illness

The so-called mentally ill form an extremely heterogeneous class of persons, but two sub-groups are typically differentiated: the 'severely mentally ill' and people with 'common mental disorders'. Although there is no clear dividing line, the former are likely to be seen as showing a greater lack of the tools for acting reasonably and with insight. They may, for instance, have experiences of an alien and imposed nature that take the form of altered states of consciousness. The person concerned may have little or no sense that they have played a part in willing them. Consequently, an illness explanation comes naturally. By contrast, so-called 'common mental disorders' are more likely to be attributed to 'psychological' (willed and modifiable) causes rather than the imposition of illness. The onus for resolving them is more firmly placed on the individual. A person is aware that something that they believe, do, or feel is irrational or out of their control despite their endeavours and self-admonishments. They have no difficulty in taking another's point of view and can usually see the desirability of changing (or concealing) some aspect of their behaviour. In essence, they fully acknowledge ownership and would agree with Szasz that even if they were to receive a diagnosis of mental illness, they would be morally accountable for resolving their problem. However, despite feeling personally responsible, a solution to their problem eludes them. Attempts to change may have made matters worse. The phrase 'neurotic conflict' refers to the self-defeating quality of worthy but failed attempts to change a woeful state of affairs. If the failure relates to an important area of life, their loss of control may induce a sense of shame or guilt.

The norms for judging a person's acts and their capacity to deal with a woe clearly vary greatly across cultures, historical periods, situations, and a person's age, status, and other characteristics. Shared norms are by definition internalised, and consequently, people may censure themselves, judging that they are 'abnormal' or 'failing to cope' (Thoits, 1985). One purpose of a psychiatric manual of disorders is to set out thresholds for what is considered to be the norm against which a person can be judged to have a mental health problem. When a norm is not shared, a person may reject the idea that their deviation warrants censure. For instance, there is a minority opinion that society is 'insane' and that 'madness' is a gift (Farber, 2012).

The 'hard cases' of so-called mental illness.

In the uncompromising language of sociology, mental illness is a form of deviancy attributable to mental or behavioural disorder. People are labelled as deviant when their behaviour affects or offends others and is unresponsive to attempts to induce conformity. Family, friends, or employers may perceive a need for 'treatment' or even hospitalisation. This form of labelling is, of course, made easier by the existence of an official set of disorders into which a person's behaviour can be fitted.

The other major class of deviancy is reserved for people who commit criminal offences. The two groups overlap. A high proportion of prisoners have either received treatment for a 'mental health problem' in the year prior to their sentence or they meet diagnostic criteria for mental illness while in prison (Prison Reform Trust, 2017). Cohen (1985) refers to 'hard' and 'soft' deviants, the former requiring firm (occasionally involuntary) social interventions. Soft deviants are those who are responsive to social sanctions; they may recognise the need to change and want help, or they are thought likely to respond to rehabilitation or therapy.

The State is primarily concerned with the 'hard cases' of so-called severe and persistent mental illness. The Mental Health Act 1983, amended 2007 (UK Government, 2007), defines a mental disorder as 'any disorder or disability of mind'. In principle, this tautology allows mental disorder to be whatever the State wants it to be. In practice, lawyers rely on psychiatric expertise, and the power of psychiatry resides in the performance of this role. Unlawful deviance due to so-called mental illness is differentiated from ordinary crime on the grounds that, with the latter, it must be established that there was *intent* for the criminal act to be committed, and that the act was *voluntarily* wrongful. A lawyer might argue that 'intent' cannot be demonstrated by reason of mental disorder, and that a person is therefore unfit to stand trial. Furthermore, when a person's ability to think rationally and act accordingly is called into question, it may be assumed (rightly or wrongly) that there is a risk that the person will cause harm to others in future. This reasoning can then be employed to justify a diagnosis of mental illness and compulsory hospital or community treatment. Thus, the law is not reserved only for people who have already acted in a threatening way and pose an obvious risk.

The Mental Capacity Act (2005) applies to people whose ability to think and act reasonably is questionable. It sets out principles for judging a person's capacity to understand and make a decision based on relevant information. Although its application is not contentious in many circumstances, this may not be the case with so-called mental illness. The Mental Health Act can, in fact, trump the Mental Capacity Act (Spandler and Anderson, 2015: 17). For instance, a person may have mental capacity in the sense of appreciating the pros and cons of taking psychoactive medication and be capable of making a decision about it. Nonetheless, this form of treatment can be imposed involuntarily. The 2007 amendment to the Mental Health Act introduced Community Treatment Orders, which are a form of conditional release from psychiatric inpatient care. The eligible patient must continue to take medication and agree to be monitored by a mental health professional. Their refusal to do so raises all of the expected dilemmas surrounding the use of a concept of mental illness to justify social control – that is, whether the policy is intended to be therapeutic for the person concerned or whether it is designed instead to reduce the perception of risk to the public. It can be difficult for a professional to remain helpful in a constructive (and non-coercive) manner when a person's right to freely make a decision about treatment can be ignored (Morgan and Felton, 2013).

Despite the humanistic foundations of Western society, it seems quite capable of inspiring subtle forms of coercion. Friedli and Stearn (2015) make out a case that welfare policies have constructed a psychological ideal that links unemployment to psychological deficit. The coercive element comes in by linking eligibility for social security benefits with various activities that are intended to modify attitudes, beliefs, and personality. This may include engaging in mandatory unpaid labour for its 'improving' effect. The underlying assumption is that unemployment is the result of personal failure and psychological deficit. Although allegations of mental unfitness do not imply a diagnosis of mental illness, they certainly border on doing so.

One recent government policy initiative aroused vigorous criticism and street protests. This was a decision to locate a therapy service in job centres for the unemployed. A Government manifesto of 2015 had stated that claimants who 'refuse a recommended treatment' may have their benefits reduced (Callard and Stearn, 2015). A letter of protest from 442 psychotherapists, counsellors, and academics appeared in a national newspaper (*The Guardian*, 2015). The policy proposal led five national organisations representing the interests of psychologists, counsellors and psychotherapists to request meetings with Government officials to seek reassurances. Two of their main worries were about people being coerced into therapy (or face sanctions), and human rights concerns about privacy and confidentiality.

The key to success in most forms of individual psychotherapy is to clarify what a person's problems are and what they can do to overcome them. The merest hint that this kind of therapy is covert coercion, with financial penalties for failing to engage in it, violates the ethical standards of all professional psychotherapy organisations. The prescription of a pharmaceutical drug is not always accompanied by a diligent search into the causes of a problem, but one can imagine the uproar if welfare claimants were required to take medication in order to receive their benefits.

'Soft cases' of so-called mental illness

Discussion of mental illness by social scientists is weighted towards the 'hard cases'. In reality, the soft cases comprise the majority of people who are potentially 'diagnosable'. However, the soft cases may not have been referred to secondary care where they could be officially diagnosed. The results of a UK survey (NHS, 2015) found that 6 per cent of men and 7 per cent of women reported taking psychoactive medication or engaging in therapy even though they did not claim to have experienced a mental health problem in the previous twelve months. It seems that even without a diagnostic label, a considerable number of people use medication or seek therapy. It is possible that some survey respondents were taking medication as a form of prophylaxis or they feared the return of 'symptoms' (or withdrawal effects) on stopping it. As regards antidepressants, there appears to be an accumulating proportion of people who, once started on them, decide to continue with medication indefinitely, and this can partially account for the rising number of annual prescriptions (Moore et al., 2009). Another indication that 'soft cases' of so-called mental illness predominate is the fact that work stress appears to be the main reason for people to visit a general practitioner (CIPD, 2011). Work stress may not result in a psychiatric diagnosis, but psychoactive medication is often prescribed in an attempt to manage it.

Seeking help for an assortment of woes, problems, or stressful situations is now commonplace and does not imply 'deviancy' in a strong sense. However, when a person formulates their problem as a disorder, it implies indoctrination into a concept of mental illness. The rising number of prescriptions for psychoactive drugs (HSCIC, 2015) suggests that medication for so-called 'common mental disorders' constitutes the backbone of present-day mental health services. Given a lack of alternatives, a medical route may be the only way a person can signal a difficulty and access a service. Taking a psychoactive drug might not be perceived as coercive, but it can be interpreted as a means by which deviance from social norms is managed.

Given that it is now so common for a person to seek help for a problem, it is not surprising that attempts are made to normalise 'mental illness' itself. In some cases, people formerly regarded as mentally ill have now come to be viewed simply as 'different'. Their behaviour has been de-medicalised. Certain differences between people are treated as acceptable examples of human diversity. Even one of the cardinal signs of madness, 'hearing voices in the head', has been normalised on the grounds that it is a very common phenomenon in the general population. The experience chiefly becomes distressing because of the way it is interpreted (see Chapter 8). Another normalising strategy is to attribute problems to impairments or disabilities rather than to mental illness (see Chapter 6). This removes the grounds for self-condemnation because a person is not usually regarded as being responsible for any impairment or disability they might happen to have. Rather than resorting to these normalising strategies, de-stigmatisation campaigns put forward the case that mental illness is an illness 'just like any other'. Consequently, it becomes an affliction, and not something that a person him or herself brings about through their own volition. The effect of this manoeuvre is to downplay the role of social processes that may have caused the woe while at the same time upholding the illness myth.

Critics of medicalisation sometimes choose a replacement term for mental illness that similarly de-emphasises its relationship to a process of social control. Beresford (2013a) refers to madness and distress, Pilgrim and McCranie (2013) to madness and misery, and Crombey, Harper and Reavey (2013) simply to psychological distress. These replacement terms represent an attempt to be non-judgmental and to convey the idea anyone can be distressed or act in a mad way. Deviance is 'normalised' by assimilating 'mental illness' into a common vocabulary of everyday words. This strategy risks creating euphemisms for mental illness or allows the new term to conceal the role of social appraisals of a person's behaviour.

Research on the prevalence of 'mental illness', defined by self-reported 'symptoms' on questionnaires, gives the impression of a continuum of distress and underplays the labelling of certain people as disordered. Crombey and colleagues (2013) point out that there is no fixed line between the normal and abnormal. Although this is true, it remains centrally important how the line is drawn, on what basis, and according to what criteria and attributions of causality. If the concept of mental illness were to be abolished, the tendency to categorise people as socially deviant would be unlikely to disappear. A somewhat different set of criteria for 'normality' would be created, and various labels applied to people who did not meet them.

As already noted, de-stigmatisation campaigns attempt to remove the distinction between physical and mental illness, thereby removing any warrant for disapproval of the latter. Mental illness is assumed to be a natural phenomenon rather like malaria. Twinley implies that there are perspectives other than a medical one when she refers to 'a social model of mental disorder' (2014: 165). It is implied that mental disorder is a phenomenon about which social scientists could have different theories. However, if mental disorder is a myth, the function of social theory should be to explain the myth's existence rather than to assume that 'mental disorder' is itself something to be explained.

A reluctance to dispense with medical terminology can be detected in other commentaries on social policy. Sapey, Spandler, and Anderson refer to the 'medicalisation of mental illness' (2015: 4), implying that mental illness is a universal category and that medicalisation is a local (cultural) variant. Weinstein argues that social workers need 'to locate and own a model of mental health that acknowledges the importance of accurate diagnosis but is not over-reliant or dependent on medical models' (2014: 12), a narrow path that seems rather difficult to tread, and does not represent an alternative to the medical model.

To advocate abolition of the concept of mental illness, and view it as a form of mystification, is not to belittle the problems of people who are distressed, impulsive, out-of-control, bothered, or woeful for all kinds of reasons. Some people might resent receiving an illness diagnosis, but mental health workers may be forced to adopt one because it is the only way they can make a case for support (Spandler, 2014: 33). Abolishing the concept of mental illness does not mean removing a need to evaluate, intervene on, and in some cases sanction, behaviour that creates a problem for self or others. Debates about the contravention of norms would simply revolve around different criteria such as a person's agency, their human rights, the reasonableness of their desires, and their willingness and ability to change.

Sketch of a theory of 'free will'

Szasz believed in free will and personal accountability for problems in living. Consequently, he thought of therapy as an exercise in rhetoric that addressed moral issues. For him, an explanation in terms of natural causes was irrelevant unless it concerned verifiable somatic disorders. This seems to leave no room for natural science to account for either free will or problems in living. The alternative I sketch out here argues that the myth of free will serves a useful function. In brief, I suggest that the myth supplies one workable arrangement for organising human relations, and that when it fails to do so successfully, the natural sciences have a useful part to play.

It is evident that people usually manage to demonstrate free will when provided with an intelligible motive for freely choosing something they want (i.e. when not under direct external compulsion). People choose freely most of the time when others expect them to do so and when their choices are consistent with an estimate of their own powers to enact that choice. It is also evident that people are occasionally unable to choose freely despite their efforts, in which case the failure may be attributed to 'psychopathology'. In these instances, the foundational assumptions of the myth of free will are not supported. However, if a belief in the myth, and its efficacious functioning, depend on optimal conditions for its acquisition in childhood, occasional failures to act upon it can be expected. Any natural causal theory that is in a position to predict these failures is strengthened as a valid scientific explanation of their occurrence.

The philosopher Schlick (1939) offered an early deterministic theory of free will. He avoided metaphysical questions about the truth of determinism and focused instead on how people actually acquire the ability to be responsible for their own acts. His idea was simply that a child learns to be responsible through the judicious application of reward and punishment for choosing the moral and/or reasonable/expected action. In other words, it is a product of social influence, chiefly parenting and education. These external influences are subsequently internalised so that a person feels responsible and acts accordingly. At this point, any transgression induces a sense of self-reproach.

Schlick emphasised the *judicious* application of reward and punishment, although the process of judging others need not be conscious or deliberate. It is directed towards a *person* who is acting independently of influences that would otherwise compel a certain response. It is clear that an adult human being is being held to account, and one who is sufficiently socialised into the concept of responsibility (i.e. a child 'who does not know better' is not yet fully trained in this respect, and in this case, the social appraisal of conduct is tempered by the need to educate). Schlick emphasised that the social judgement is not concerned with taking account of causal influences such as a person's genes or the character of their grandparents. However, in the immediate situation in which a person's act is being evaluated, the application of praise or blame takes account of external factors that are not under a person's direct control (e.g. inebriation or an emotion of fear induced by danger). Schlick makes the indisputable point that: 'If decisions were causeless, there would be no sense in trying to influence men' (1939: 157). In his opinion, the more motives we can find for an act, the more we regard a person as responsible for it. Schlick states that 'In general we know very well how to discover the causes of conduct in the characters of our fellow men, and how to use this knowledge in the prediction of their future behaviour . . .' (ibid.: 157). This sounds rather over-optimistic but for Schlick's account to be credible, there must exist sufficient consistency (i.e. normativity) in social responding for a sense of responsibility and its limits to be acquired.

As regards the *feeling* of being responsible for one's acts, Schlick argued that the subjective feeling coincides with the objective judgement. In other words, 'the person blamed or condemned is conscious of the fact that he was "rightly" taken to account' (ibid.: 151). In addition to a person being seen as the true doer of an act must also be added 'the awareness that he did it "independently" on his own initiative' (ibid.: 154). On Schlick's account, the consciousness of freedom is a kind of felicitous delusion that is self-fulfilling because the freedom we ascribe to ourselves informs the evaluative judgements we apply to others – which guarantees their 'freedom' also because it is the means by which agency is acquired. The account is credible because it is consistent with what we know about the effects of inadequate parenting or abuse in early childhood that can lead to the loss of a normal sense of agency. It may lead, for example, to an adult being under-assertive, feeling overly responsible, or conversely, acting with a sense of entitlement (e.g. de Carvalho et al., 2015; Hengartner et al., 2015; Huh et al., 2015).

Schlick did not seem to appreciate the difficulty of applying his ideas to the behaviour of the non-average person who does not act as expected:

> In the case of a person who is mentally ill, we do not consider him free with respect to those acts in which the disease expresses itself, because we view the illness as a disturbing factor which hinders the normal functioning of his natural tendencies.
>
> *Schlick, 1939: 151*

This is a neat summing-up of the social function performed by the concept of mental illness. Schlick does not offer an independent definition of mental illness, and so his statement is an example of circular reasoning. It amounts to saying that whatever removes our normal volitional powers can be explained by mental illness (the evidence for which is the loss of our volitional powers).

Schlick's employment of the concept of mental illness to explain why some people are stripped of their power of agency has been criticised by Pickard (2015). She points out that most workers in the field of mental health do not think of agency in this all-or-none fashion, and do not attribute a person's failure to change to the presence or absence of mental illness. As Pickard puts it, the agency of clients/patients/service-users is only impaired relative to the norm. In her view, deviant behaviour should be classified as an act implying intent, and therefore a behaviour over which a person can exert some control. In the case of acts associated with so-called mental illness, we might desist from blaming a person (knowing it to be ineffective), but still hold a person responsible and capable of showing a willingness to change. For example, from the fact that an addict can control their compulsive habit under some circumstances, Pickard argues that he or she 'possesses the general ability to control their use in a broad range of circumstances' (ibid.: 148).

The assumption of a general ability (undefined) seems to overstate the case. Rather, control is possible under certain circumstances, justifying the belief that control could possibly be extended to new circumstances. This is a judgement that may or may not be borne out by experience. If it is not, or if some previously undetected and powerful causal influence is discovered, one might as well say that the person lacks agency (with regard to their particular problem) in any meaningful sense. Pickard suggests that the 'general ability' just mentioned could be construed metaphorically as a faculty of willpower, acting rather like a muscle (Muraven and Baumeister, 2000). Willpower, according to this account, is seen as an ability for conscious and sustained effort. However, if at some point willpower fails, what are we to conclude? We can agree with Pickard that a belief that a person's behaviour is caused by an illness or disease is likely to have a disempowering effect because it would diminish motivation to exercise whatever willpower a person possesses.

Pickard's argument blurs the meaning of voluntary to include 'potentially voluntary'. Her analysis corresponds to Szasz's adoption of the distinction between causes and reasons (which also translates for him into physical illness versus so-called mental illness). Pickard states that where executive function is lost due to a physical state, 'behaviour approximates an automatic reflex' (2015: 156). An alternative to this position, consistent with natural causation, is to abandon the assumption that 'naturally caused' means 'illness' (or, indeed, any other special category of 'automatic process' in the body). This implies that it is necessary to reinterpret the cause/reason dichotomy so that it can be reconciled with the natural causation of all behaviour.

As Schlick argues, the distinction between voluntary and involuntary rests ultimately upon a social evaluation in relation to particular circumstances. Although the categories of behaviour referred to as 'naturally caused' and 'reasoned' must have some different causal antecedents, these are not at all easy to identify. Even the eye-blink reflex has voluntary and learned elements and has been classified into different types (Rasmussen and Jirenhed, 2017). In fact, acts regarded as involuntary could have many complex causes, including the effects of the deliberate social appraisal of an act, whether delivered by others or oneself. If Schlick is correct that free will is acquired and maintained as a result of education and the social appraisal of conduct, there is no reason to discount the possibility that mal-education and 'unreasonable' social appraisals can result in conduct labelled as 'mental illness'.

The judgement of an act as 'voluntary' depends in part on what is regarded as 'normal' (i.e. socially approved) in the circumstances. From the standpoint of natural causation, it is hardly credible to suppose that voluntary and involuntary acts have neatly segregated causes. In any case, the existence of voluntary behaviour would be implausible without involuntary processes to support it (Roessler, 2003; Hallam, 2009: 191–214). Moreover, an act that is done initially freely and for a good reason may become a strong habit and eventually develop into an involuntary compulsion.

Consider, as an illustration of social appraisal, the fact that mothers are not viewed as showing compulsive (involuntary) love for their babies, even though they would find it extremely difficult to alter their habitual behaviour. Rather, mothers who freely volunteer that they do not feel motherly (but continue to mother their babies) are often regarded as 'pathological', even though their non-motherly feelings are not experienced as compulsive. There may, of course, be certain responses that are always judged to be reflexive (and are therefore experienced as involuntary), but both simple and complexly determined behaviour share the capacity to be influenced in such a way as to be perceived as freely chosen or, contrariwise, imposed (determined).

Abolition of the concept of mental illness would only rule out certain kinds of assumption about natural causes, namely, the sorts of unsubstantiated criteria put forward to claim that a mental illness exists. In textbooks of medicine, psychiatric disorders, if they are mentioned at all, are included under neurology (e.g. Goldman and Schafer, 2015). It is assumed that 'mental illness' is caused by a neurological disease (which in certain cases it might be). However, ruling out neural pathology does not mean that so-called mental illness is not mediated by natural causes.

The standard interpretation given to the natural causation of 'mental illnesses' is that they have to be traced back to a stand-alone brain – that neuroscience will provide the key to future progress. This belief does not do justice to natural causation at a societal level of analysis. For example, emergent processes in human behaviour (emergent at the individual or collective level) can be assumed to be examples of natural causation (Elder-Vass, 2010). Brain-based theories of the causes of so-called mental illness seem to have been led astray by religious and philosophical beliefs about human nature (Hallam, 2012). This leads to a search for the origins of 'willpower' in the brain because this organ is understood to be the seat of the mind (originally the soul with all its God-given faculties).

On Schlick's account, a person's ability to distinguish between what are normatively classified as voluntary and involuntary acts is necessary in order to judge them and assign moral responsibility. Mental health professionals in non-coercive settings work on the assumption that a person intends to change, and all parties presume that change is possible. However, a person's intention to exercise responsibility does not guarantee that change will occur. In any case, psychosocial formulations of problems frequently distribute responsibility to other people as well, for instance, to a past or present abuser, who could be a parent (Pilgrim, 2016). Therefore, in theorising a person's responsibility for making a change (from a natural science perspective), the analysis can extend far beyond the identified client/service-user. In fact, a person might be invited to consider the causal influence of others (or cultural assumptions that they endorse) in order to gain a better appreciation of their ownership of a problem. This may result in re-assigning responsibility to other people. The purpose is not to remove personal responsibility but to relieve a person of unreasonable blame or guilt in line with common assumptions about what it is 'reasonable' for any person to be responsible for.

The role of volition in therapy is therefore complex. Clients/service-users frequently choose to be influenced by interventions over which they have no direct control. This clearly applies to any medication that affects the brain. However, in re-skilling and other re-learning methods, a person also submits to a method whose outcome they cannot predict with certainty. For this reason, there are ethical controls on false representation of the benefits to be had from applying any therapy technique.

Reconciling natural causation and personal responsibility for a 'mental health problem'

When a person acknowledges the existence of a problem, there is a rather subtle relationship between the self that wills to change and that part of the self that is externalised as 'the problem'. This has been well described by Rego (2004), drawing upon the writings of the philosopher Harry Frankfurt (1988). A person who is so enmeshed with their problem that they cannot perceive what it is must first externalise it in some way in order to be able to address it. Typically, this leads to discord between their frustration or unhappiness and their uncertain ability to do anything about it. By dissociating that part of themselves which constitutes the problem from the self that chooses to overcome it, a person is able to reflect and employ their agency from a new standpoint. The essential idea drawn from Frankfurt is that there are first order, second order, and third order thoughts or desires. For example, a person might want to smoke, want not to smoke, and also think that it is idle to contemplate whether or not to give up smoking (third order), given the strength of their addiction. A person at some point decides which attitude to adopt and withdraws allegiance from the other options. This effectively ends the appeal to higher order thoughts or desires even though they may remain available for reflection. According to Frankfurt, a person's decision to adopt an attitude to a problem contributes to the way they define their identity. As Rego summarises his position: 'The patient can now treat him- or herself in a manner of speaking. She or he can relate to the problem at hand in a quasi-third person style by appreciating its characteristics and interacting with them in a prescribed manner' (2004: 316).

The medical model of woes is also a form of objective distancing. A bodily symptom can be viewed from a second order perspective, assuming that the illness is not an advanced dementia that precludes reflection and memory. The chief problem with the view that mental illness defines what a person is (e.g. unstable, neurotic, depressed, deluded, etc.) is that it discourages the employment of higher order perspectives. The biomedical model assumes that what a person has to deal with has already been decided. In this way, it reduces the options open to them.

It is well documented that people go through various stages when they entertain making a change and then act upon it. Prochaska, DiClemente, and Norcross (1992) describe the stages as pre-contemplation, contemplation, action, and maintenance. This sounds like a well-thought out reflective process, but the experiences that prompt reflection have a complex relationship with a sense of agency and self. A person's unwanted experience may already be 'external' if it lacks a normal sense of ownership, and consequently it may be perceived as an intrusion that is attributed to alien forces. The problem is still one's own ('this is happening to me') but a sense of agency is lost, i.e. some alien process or person is causing it to happen (Gallagher, 2004). There are also lesser degrees of a loss of agency, e.g. 'I feel compelled to think certain thoughts', or 'I can't stop myself having this impulse (even though I know I won't act upon it)'. All of this suggests that a sense of agency is, at times, a fragile construction. From a medical perspective, unwanted experiences interpreted as symptoms have been attributed to neural dysfunctions, but this still leaves a person in the position of trying to make sense of them. The attempt may produce bizarre results, but as Gallagher notes in relation to a diagnosis of schizophrenia: 'Some level of the schizophrenic person's thought must remain unaffected by the disruption of agency, otherwise she would be unable to complain of alien movements, thoughts, or voices' (2004: 98). Recent evidence suggests that alien experiences are potentially understandable in terms of prior (historical) traumatic childhood events (Read et al., 2005). In pre-modern societies, unusual experiences, such as hearing hallucinated voices, were not necessarily seen as abnormal phenomena, and other interpretations (e.g. the actions of gods or spirits) were more readily available (Leudar and Thomas, 2000).

The concept of mental illness mystifies by explaining a woe as something that is caused by a bodily disorder. The alternative outlined by Rego (2004) is to transform a distressing experience into a phenomenon with which a person can grapple as an objectified element within their total personality. Of course, a person still has to contemplate making a change and to act upon it. This raises the question of whether it is reasonable to assign responsibility (to the affected person or to others) and whether the parties actually have the freedom and power to act. At the two ends of a continuum of power, we have Szasz's 'free will' and, at the other, the social/materialist position of authors such as Smail (2005) and the Midlands Psychology Group (MPG, 2014).

Smail argues that 'there is no such thing as an autonomous individual' (2005: 46), and he regards the client/patient as a victim who lacks the resources to combat external power in all its forms. He thinks that a therapist can, at best, support, comfort, and possibly help to articulate the state of affairs in which the person finds herself. This view seems to underestimate the extent to which anyone described as mentally ill can exercise their agency and powers of reflection. Szasz's position (that people by default are morally accountable for all of their acts) errs in the opposite direction. As Schlick (1939) theorised, the power of agency and rational self-governance are acquired in childhood, and in Western societies this learning is non-optional. Few concessions are made to adults however adverse their early education or later social environment has been. Autonomy and the ability to change are our default assumptions even though their fit to reality is approximate. Some people simply take their own life when change seems impossible. In the UK population survey cited above, 4 per cent of men and 7 per cent of women reported either self-harm or suicide attempts (NHS, 2015). Suicide is the leading cause of death among young people (WHO, 2001).

The Midlands Psychology Group (MPG, 2014: 124), like Rose (1999), are suspicious of the ideology of autonomy (free will), and follow Michel Foucault in seeing it as a product of the social, historical, and material circumstances in which we find ourselves. They maintain that 'distress is not the consequence of inner flaws or weaknesses'. If that is so, it excludes entirely any question of moral accountability (MPG, 2014: 123). However, MPG accepts that people often view their distress in moral terms and they point out that 'experience and explanation are two very different things' (ibid.: 124). I take this to mean that a belief in personal autonomy is, from their standpoint, a form of false consciousness, a position similar to the one I outlined earlier that 'free will' has mythical elements. However, a belief in free will is not 'false' in the sense implied by MPG because it can be cultivated and rendered effective. In support of their position, MPG point to a correlation between woes and a person's level of material resources, class, gender, and other forms of social inequality.

The consciousness of freedom may be false in the sense that it reflects a political ideology (i.e. it is mythical and constructed rather than a natural endowment), but the fact remains that we live in a society founded on a belief in autonomy and freedom of choice. In the absence of a worked-out political alternative, any criticism of the status-quo acceptance of autonomy lacks credibility and force. Although social arrangements reliant on a belief in free will can lead to manifestly unfair outcomes, people are unlikely to prefer to be governed through more transparent forms of coercion or to want to return to a pre-modern belief in malign forces. It does a client or service-user no favours (given the social contingencies they have to face) to regard them as a victim who has little power to resist or change. In fact, this attitude could be said to reinforce the social messages they have already received about powerlessness.

In practice, MPG reverts to a belief that therapy and/or medication can foster a person's reasoning and agency, e.g. 'help people make better use of the powers and resources already available to them', 'draw attention to unrecognised resources', and 'explicitly support people to cease viewing themselves as 'the problem' (2014: 134). They observe that clients particularly value listening, understanding, and respectfulness. 'Respect' is as much a product of a political philosophy of autonomy and volition as it is an ideological support for a welfare policy that is engineered to make the individual feel personally responsible for their woes. Rose (1999), Smail (2005: iv) and Foucault (see Oksala, 2005) all seem to endorse a concept of freedom that goes beyond, and is incompatible with, their main theoretical presuppositions. The paradox is that a sense of freedom is both acquired and maintained as a consequence of being exposed to external sanctions, including punishment. At the same time, our sense of freedom seems to include an element of non-restraint whose source remains elusive.

The role of the concept of mental illness in policies that stress personal accountability

When the status of being a free moral agent is assigned by default, for an adult to claim otherwise requires special pleading. However, because the process of acquiring agency is largely invisible, there may be a failure to respond sympathetically when a person does not act according to common norms of what is reasonable and morally justifiable. Society can adopt at least two positions to reconcile deviant behaviour with the presumption that a person should be accountable for their acts. The first is to suppose that the presence of a so-called mental illness removes the obligation or explains the deviation (see earlier discussion). The second position amounts to various degrees of disapproval and censure combined with re-education. This response comes naturally when a person does not demonstrate 'strength of character' or ignores the feelings and wishes of others. Incomprehension applies especially to people given a diagnosis of personality disorder. Their non-conformity is usually episodic and, being unexpected, it may catch others off-guard. As a Department of Health information booklet explains it: 'We may find ourselves feeling uncharacteristically frustrated with someone, or eager to help and "rescue" them from their difficulties, or feeling we have to tip-toe around them for fear of provoking them' (Tavistock and Portman NHS Foundation Trust, 2017: 4).

Therapists who work with people given this diagnosis have to train themselves to suppress their spontaneous responses of annoyance or disapproval (Linehan, 1993). The 'natural' reaction to someone who violates the norms of social interaction points to the function that these reactions serve in enforcing social conformity.

In other words, disapproval or censure, besides being social judgements, can be understood as having a natural causal effect on a person's behaviour. Contrariwise, a person's resolve, and consequently their power of agency, can be strengthened by praise and encouragement. In a society founded on the concept of a person as a free agent, we have no option but to approve or disapprove when we feel it is justified. If we did not do so, the functional integrity of this social arrangement would presumably break down.

Abolishing the concept of mental illness would not remove a need to evaluate, and in some cases attempt to modify or sanction, behaviour that creates a problem for self or others. Debates about deviancy would simply revolve around different criteria. These are likely to include the probable success of non-coercive measures, human rights, and risk to other people, in so far as this can be ascertained. At present, society's response to behaviour that confounds social expectations often gives out a mixed message about responsibility and 'illness'. This is nicely illustrated in the journals of a man diagnosed with schizophrenia in the 1960s who spent most of his adult life in psychiatric hospitals (Hallam and Bender, 2011). On the one hand he was diagnosed as ill, accepted his diagnosis, swallowed his pills, and was puzzled by experiences that were clearly puzzling:

> The delusion to which I am referring is simply this. I was hearing voices, and for a long time assumed them to be some form of hallucination. But, just as a strong man can be broken with the dripping tap torture in five minutes used during the last war, so these voices – repeating everything I said and making comments (sometimes obscene) eventually drove me into the false belief that they were real.
>
> *Hallam and Bender, 2011: 225*

On the other hand (and in that era), he had to contribute to the cost of hospital care out of his welfare payments and to deal with his own tax affairs. He was assumed to be capable of taking advantage of industrial rehabilitation and to find a job. At various times, he was regarded simultaneously as 'lazy' and 'ill'. When being interviewed for a job (while residing in hospital), he said that he suffered from 'mild schizophrenia'. This lost him the job and his mental welfare officer was completely furious with him for having mentioned it (ibid.: 141). For this young man, the concept of mental illness confused what was already a puzzling state of mind, and he received mixed messages about how to act responsibly. By mentioning 'mild schizophrenia' at his job interview, he was being quite reasonable in his own eyes, either deliberately torpedoing his chances of getting a job or alerting his potential employer that he could not be relied upon 100 per cent of the time. This illustration is taken from a different era, but there is little reason to suppose that mixed messages about personal responsibility have not persisted with respect to the 'mentally ill'.

The position taken by professionals engaged in therapy or rehabilitation is to encourage people to be more responsible for their actions so that they conform more and deviate less. For instance, interventions are presented as interpersonal strategies designed to enhance responsible self-governance (Rose, 1999). To be consistent with the myth of free will, engagement with them has to be seen as freely and voluntarily undertaken. As this is expressed in the ethical code of the British Psychological Society, all practising psychologists must 'value the dignity and worth of all persons, with sensitivity to the dynamics of perceived authority or influence over clients, and with particular regard to people's rights including those of privacy and self determination' (BPS, 2009: 9). In practice, this means that any practitioner must obtain informed consent, keep confidential notes securely, and register as a data controller with the Information Commissioner's Office. The function of this code of ethics is primarily to protect a service user's/client's human rights. The aim of non-coercive methods is to return a person to a state of self-determination (free will).

'Responsibilizing' welfare policies are a counterpart to a political concept of freedom. Rose sees them as a disguised form of social control (Rose, 1999: 54). The objective is to foster freedom by appearing to reinforce the positive value of autonomy while in practice it serves to strengthen conformity to norms that are mostly promoted by the State, by experts, and by mental health entrepreneurs. As Rose points out, it is not only governments but also radical political thinkers who have advocated a style of existence in which a person works upon him/herself in the name of freedom. Authenticity and self-expression are usually celebrated. Rose sees the policies of advanced liberal governments as having developed from the aim of 'freeing' people in the realms of the market, civil society, and the family: 'The private conduct of free citizens was to be civilised by equipping them with languages and techniques of self-understanding and self-mastery' (ibid.: 69). Expressed differently, the good citizen 'would govern themselves through introspection, foresight, calculation, judgement and according to certain ethical norms' (ibid.: 78). With regard to policies on health, 'individuals are addressed on the assumption that they want to be healthy, and enjoined to freely seek out the ways of living most likely to promote their own health' (ibid.: 86). Rose believes that this has encouraged a view of health as consumption, where choice is influenced by experts, by entrepreneurs of the health market, and by advertising.

At first glance, a consumerist approach to mental health is congenial to the policies of advanced liberalism. However, there are some rather obvious mismatches with reality on the ground. As a consumer, a person is only relatively autonomous because she/he is not an isolated agent who can choose regardless of the interests of family, friends, or employer. In any case, a person might be mystified as to what choices are available to them. It would be stretching the facts to say that most people are informed consumers as far as their own mental health is concerned.

There have been moves in the UK to give greater personal control and choice over care received. This has taken the form of direct State funding of a personal budget for people with long-term health or social care needs. The budget is an agreed amount of money that is planned in conjunction with a health professional. This is only a limited form of consumer choice because there is a lengthy application procedure and spending has to be approved in the light of explicit goals. As expressed by the charity, Rethink: 'It can be difficult to find the balance between someone being well enough to make decisions about what they need whilst also having severe enough needs to meet high eligibility criteria' (Rethink, n.d.).

The demand for a personalised service came initially from service-users who wanted to have more say in what was being offered to them (Beresford, 2013b; Weinstein, 2014: 12). This fits with a consumerist philosophy but the government decided to impose this model for whomever it is eligible, whether or not it was wanted or appropriate. *Genuine* consumer choice is rather limited within statutory services. For example, service-users are rarely able to choose their key worker or therapist.

In practice, it is mental health and social welfare managers who are the consumers and make decisions about how to spend their resources. They need suppliers who offer products that can be operationally defined and counted. The managerial approach is accompanied by a drive to reduce costs and increase the predictability of operating procedures. Problems are specified in standard ways, functions are compartmentalised, and there is strict control over processes, such as the permissible number of sessions. Uniform outcome measures are adopted, allegedly for the purposes of quality control. None of this is conducive to consumer choice. To allow genuine consumer choice would mean providing a wider range of options and alternative ways of conceptualising problems that take greater account of their uniqueness. Target setting with simple measures encourages a distortion of good practice, such as maximising throughput using a narrow definition of outcome. Examples of these effects in community mental health services are given by Moth (2014) and Brammer (2014), and for counselling and psychotherapy in the National Health Service by Proctor (2015).

Rationalisation occurred earlier in the United States and with some clearly undesirable consequences. Managed Care Organisations (HMOs) and private health insurers have adopted psychiatric diagnosis as the basis for approved funding. Cushman and Gilford point out what a profound influence this is:

> Whoever controls the delivery of mental health care – by determining such things as the definition of mental disorder, triage criteria, and the nature and length of proper treatment – inevitably and deeply affects society-wide understanding of health and illness, abnormality and healing, the possibilities and limits of human nature and thus what is believed to be proper and good.
>
> *Cushman and Gilford, 2000: 985*

They note that the consumer taking advantage of their insurance scheme may have little choice on what is offered. Some HMOs 'require their clients to sign treatment contracts that state that non-compliance can be grounds from dismissal from the HMO treatment benefit'. Alternatively, in the face of non-compliance, they may 'invoke a more pejorative diagnosis' such as personality disorder that is not reimbursable (ibid.: 988).

The distortion of a concept of mental health to force it in line with an aim of decreasing dependency on welfare is evident in UK government publications (see Chapter 8). Many service users/survivors who took part in a recent consumer survey (Beresford et al., 2016) felt that the idea of 'recovery from illness' had been subverted by government policy. For them, it had come to be defined in terms of people coming off benefits and getting a job, rather than improving their life chances.

Rose is sceptical of 'responsibilizing' forms of social control but he does express an opinion, rather sketchily articulated, on 'genuine' responsibility and freedom of choice. He mentions volunteers with a radical agenda who operate outside bureaucratic structures. He also notes that expertise is sometimes generously shared. He refers to 'bereavement counsellors who cluster around events from the illness of a child to the experience of a plane crash' (Rose, 1999: 91). Having argued that freedom is relative, historical, technical, and tied up with power and subordination, Rose is led to abandon the idea that 'subjectivity is privileged as the authentic and natural locus of moral autonomy' (ibid.: 95). If his were to be a complete account of subjectivity, a person would have no compass at all to give them a sense of direction, apart from the advice of experts and State regulators. Nevertheless, given the corner into which he has driven himself, Rose does ask how we can 'orient ourselves to the value of freedom' (ibid.: 95). His tentative answer is 'to value all stratagems, tactics, and practices that enhance human beings' capacities to act' (ibid.: 97). The values underlying Rose's position are therefore unclear. He would 'evaluate practices in terms of the extent to which they accord those caught up within them the capacity to judge, accept or transform the practices that subjectify them . . . to be open, inventive, and questioning' (ibid.). These sentiments, which could certainly be understood as a clarion call to anyone seeking alternatives to present mental health services, seem to give back what he has already taken away theoretically.

Rationale for a mental health service

The assumption that mental illness 'exists', and needs a mental health service to deal with it, creates an expectation that the State should attend to everyone's 'mental ill-health'. However, it is quite evident that physical health and mental health do not receive equal attention or funding. This is understandable inasmuch as the circumstances to which mental illness refers are elastic and unquantifiable. Abandoning the concept would at least allow a cooler appraisal of the likely causes and promising solutions for each type of woe, leading to a better appreciation of where responsibility should lie – whether with the individual, with the community, with the State, or with these sources of agency acting together.

So-called mental illnesses are somewhat more reactive to events than many physical illnesses. The cause of a physical illness might, of course, be accidental or unforeseen but once diagnosed, plans can usually be put in place to deal with future contingencies. Treatment can sometimes be delayed. For so-called mental illness, immediate and timely action is often crucial. Even for those people who are regarded as having a 'long-term mental illness', unforeseen crises can arise which require immediate attention. Weinstein (2014: 22–24) gives the example of a man who disturbed his neighbours in a community setting and shows how the crisis needed to be understood (and assessed) from at least half a dozen angles, each with a different implication for the urgency (or otherwise) of taking action. Even for a person who is generally functioning well, it makes no sense at all to wait weeks or months for an appointment with a mental health professional. Prompt action is more likely to lead to a resolution, allowing a person to return to work or cope with a crisis. A person might have reflected for some time before seeking help but, even then, the time window for acting and making a change is usually narrow.

Although the State is necessarily involved in responding to at least a proportion of people in distress, there are several objections to framing this social obligation as a response to mental illness:

(1) The accountability of the State and the individual is not at present transparent or made explicit (i.e. there is mystification about causes and responsibilities).
(2) Assigning responsibility to the State for the rectification of woes (e.g. the provision of treatment for 'mental illness') runs the risk of downplaying the role (and human rights) of the individual. It should be possible to devise other interventions that are less coercive and permit a person to overcome their woe through their own efforts or jointly with others.
(3) If each type of woe has characteristic causes and needs to be resolved in a variety of ways, there is little to be gained by assuming that 'mental illnesses' have anything much in common. The 'mental health system' is to a large extent already a collection of unrelated activities and functions.
(4) The response of mental health services is often inordinately slow and inflexible, and being slow or untimely, any intervention is less likely to be effective. In many cases, it is the police service that deals with emergencies.

Recent recommendations to the UK Government from a Mental Health Task Force (MHTF) (DOH, 2016) include a call for parity between physical and mental health services, and don't hesitate to inflate the need:

> We know that the scale of unmet mental health need is significant – hundreds of thousands of people go untreated each year at a cost of billions of pounds to our society and the economy . . . The whole NHS plays a role in preventing mental health problems and caring for people who suffer them.
>
> *DOH, 2016: 66*

That there are unmet needs cannot be questioned, but the language of treatment, caring, and suffering may be inappropriate. People may not want to be labelled as mentally ill or receive 'treatment' from the State. To seek help or advice from this source places a person in the position of a supplicant. A supplicant is defined as someone who asks humbly for something from a god or person in authority. For a person whose problems may well have originated in coercive parenting or abuse of various kinds, a sense of agency may not be best cultivated by providing 'treatment'.

The MHTF implicitly confirms the one-down position of a service-user when they state: 'This is critical in enabling people with mental health problems to play a more active role in making choices about all aspects of their care, based on a more equal and collaborative relationship between the person and professional(s)' (ibid.: 43).

Summary

The illness myth accounts for why some people act in ways that disturb others and why they demonstrate an inability to solve their own woes. The myth can be viewed as a form of mystification that attributes the reasons for these failures to conform to a person's 'illness' or 'disorder'. This account de-emphasises the part played by social processes in causing and maintaining woes. The myth is supported by strategies to rename mental illness as ordinary distress or impairment. The belief that mental illness is 'just like any other illness' reinforces the myth. In effect, campaigns to de-stigmatise 'mental illness' conceal the circumstances that produce woes. One effect of abolishing the concept of mental illness would be to reveal rather than hide the significance of social appraisal and control. Abolition need not carry the implication that people should (in general) be made to feel more or less responsible for resolving their woes. The case for abolition presented above is framed within a deterministic theory of the acquisition of agency, in which 'free will' is viewed as a useful myth that serves to organise social relations. This framework is used, in turn, to throw light on the process of regaining self-control in therapy, on social policies that stress individual responsibility, and to inform a rationale for the future provision of well-being services.

References

Beresford, P. (2013a) Experiential knowledge and the reconception of madness. In: Coles, S., Keenan, S. & Diamond, B. (eds.) *Madness contested: Power and practice*, Ross-on-Wye, PCCS Books, pp.181–196.

Beresford, P. (2013b) *Personalisation, critical and radical debates in social work*. Bristol, Policy.

Beresford, P., Perring, R., Nettle, M., & Wallcraft, J. (2016) *From mental illness to a social model of madness and distress*. Published by Shaping Our Lives. Available from: www.shapingourlives.org.uk/wp-content/uploads/2016/05/FROM-MENTAL-ILLNESS-PDF-2.pdf [Accessed 12 December 2016].

BPS (2009) *Code of ethics and conduct: Guidance published by the ethics committee of the British Psychological Society*. Leicester, The British Psychological Society.

Brammer, A. (2014) Observations from the front line. In: Weinstein, J. (ed.) *Mental health: Critical and radical debates in social work*, Ferguson, I. & Lavalette, M. (series eds.). Bristol, Policy, pp.77–82.

Callard. F. & Stearn, R. (2015) Facing psychological coercion and manipulation has become a daily part of claiming benefits. *The Conversation*, 8 June. Available from: https://theconversation.com/facing-psychological-coercion-and-manipulation-has-become-a-daily-part-of-claiming-benefits 42839?utm_campaign=BACP+News%3A+June+2015&utm_source=emailCampaign&utm_medium=email&utm_content= [Accessed 10 May 2017].

CIPD (Chartered Institute of Personnel Development) (2011) *Stress and mental health at work*. London, CIPD.

Cohen, S. (1985) *Visions of social control: Crime, punishment, and classification*. Cambridge, Polity Press.

Crombey, J., Harper., D. & Reavey, P. (2013) *Psychology, mental health, and distress*. Basingstoke, Palgrave.

Cushman, P. & Gilford, P. (2000) Will managed care change our way of being? *American Psychologist*. 55, pp.985–996.

de Carvalho, H. W., Pereira, R., Frozi, J., Bisol, L. W., Ottoni, G. L. & Lara, D. R. (2015) Childhood trauma is associated with maladaptive personality traits. *Child Abuse and Neglect*. 44, pp.18–25.

Elder-Vass, D. (2010) *The causal power of social structures: Emergence, structure and agency*. Cambridge, Cambridge University Press.

Farber, S. (2012) *The spiritual gift of madness: The failure of psychiatry and the rise of the mad pride movement*. Rochester, VT, Inner Traditions.

Frankfurt, H. G. (1988) *The importance of what we care about: Philosophical essays*. Cambridge, Cambridge University Press.

Friedli, L. & Stearn, R. (2015) Positive affect as coercive strategy: Conditionality, activation and the role of psychology in UK government workfare programmes. *Medical Humanities*, 41, pp.40–47.

Gallagher, S. (2004) Agency, ownership, and alien control in schizophrenia, In: Zahavi, D., Grunbaum, T., & Parnas J. (eds.) *The structure and development of self-consciousness*. Amsterdam, John Benjamins, pp.89–104.

Goldman, L. & Schafer, A. I. (2015) *Goldman-Cecil medicine (Cecil textbook of medicine)*, 25th edn. New York, Elsevier.

Hallam, R. S. (2012) Disordered selves. *Contemporary Social Science*. 7 (2), 197–213.

Hallam, R. S. (2009) *Virtual selves, real persons: A dialogue across disciplines*. Cambridge, Cambridge University Press.

Hallam, R. S. & Bender, M. (2011) *David's box: The journals and letters of a young man diagnosed as schizophrenic, 1960–1971*. London, Polpresa Press.

Hengartner, M. P., Ajdacic-Gross, V., Rodgers, S., Müller, M. & Rössler, W. (2013) Childhood adversity in association with personality disorder dimensions: New findings in an old debate. *European Psychiatry*. 28(8), pp.476–482.

HSCIC (2015) *Prescriptions dispensed in the community in England, 2004–2014*. Health and Social Care Information Centre, 7 July. Available from: www.hscic.gov.uk [Accessed 12 December 2016].

Huh, H., Kim, S., Yu, J. J. & Chae, J. (2014) Childhood trauma and adult interpersonal relationship problems in patients with depression and anxiety disorders. *Annals of General Psychiatry*. 13, p.26. Available from: https://annals-general-psychiatry.biomedcentral.com/articles/10.1186/s12991-014-0026-y [Accessed 10 May 2017].

Leudar, I. & Thomas, P. (2000) *Voices of reason, voices of insanity: Studies of verbal hallucinations*. London, Routledge.

Linehan, M. M. (1993) *Cognitive behavioral treatment of borderline personality disorder*. New York, Guilford.

Morgan, A. & Felton, A. (2013) From constructive engagement to coerced recovery. In: Coles, S., Keenan, S. & Diamond, B. (eds.) *Madness contested: Power and practice*. Ross-on-Wye, PCCS Books, pp.56–73.

Moore, M. et al. (2009) Explaining the rise in antidepressant prescribing: A descriptive study using the general practice research database. *British Medical Journal*, 339, b3999.

Moth, R. (2014) 'Diagnosis human': Markets, targets and medicalisation in community mental health services. In Weinstein, J. (ed.) *Mental health: Critical and radical debates in social work* (series eds. Ferguson, I. & Lavalette, M.). Bristol, Policy, pp.57–61.

MPG (Midlands Psychology Group) (2013) Manifesto for a social materialist psychology of distress. In: Coles, S., Keenan, S. & Diamond. B. (eds.) *Madness contested: Power and practice*. Ross-on-Wye, PCCS Books, pp.121–140.

Muraven, M. & Baumeister, R. F. (2000) Self-regulation and depletion of resources: Does self-control resemble a muscle? *Psychological Bulletin*, 126(2), pp.247–259.

NHS (2015) *Health survey for England, 2014*. Available from: www.content.digital.nhs.uk [Accessed 10 May 2017].

Oksala, J. (2005) *Foucault on freedom*. Cambridge, Cambridge University Press.

Pickard, H. (2015) Psychopathology and the ability to do otherwise. *Philosophy and Phenomenological Research*. XC(1), pp.135–163.

Pilgrim, D. (2016) Addiction and multi-party ethical responsibility. *Clinical Psychology Forum*. 278, pp.4–7.

Pilgrim, D. & McCrainie, A. (2013) *Recovery and mental health: A critical sociological account*. Basingstoke, Palgrave.

Prison Reform Trust (2017) Mental health care in prisons. Available from: *www.prisonreformtrust.org.uk/projectsresearch/mentalhealth* [Accessed 10 May 2017].

Prochaska, J. O., DiClemente, C. C. & Norcross, J. C. (1992) In search of how people change: Applications to addictive behaviors. *American Psychologist*, 47(9), pp.1102–1114.

Proctor, G. (2015) The NHS in 2015: Still a scary possibility to come. *Healthcare Counselling & Psychotherapy Journal* (October), pp.8–16.

Rasmussen, A. & Jirenhed, D. (2017) Learning and timing of voluntary blink responses match eyeblink conditioning. *Nature: Scientific Reports*. 7, Art. 3404. Available from: https://www.nature.com/articles/s41598-017-03343-2 [Accessed 10 July 2017].

Read, J., van Os, J., Morrison, A. P. & Ross, C. A. (2005) Childhood trauma, psychosis and schizophrenia: A literature review with theoretical and clinical implications. *Acta Psychiatrica Scandinavica*. 112, pp.330–350.

Rego, M. D. (2004) Externality in psychiatry and the paradox of agency. *Philosophy, Psychology, Psychiatry*. 11(4), pp.313–321.

Rethink (n.d.) Your guide to personal budgets. Available from: https://www.rethink.org/media/829663/1%20Considering%20a%20Personal%20Budget.pdf [Accessed 10 May 2017].

Roessler, J. (2003) Intentional action and self-awareness. In: Roessler, R. & Elan, N. (eds.) *Agency and self-awareness: Issues in philosophy and psychology*. New York, Oxford University Press, pp.383–405.

Rose, N. (1999) *Powers of freedom: Reframing political thought*. Cambridge, Cambridge University Press.

Ryle, G. (1949) *The concept of mind*. London, Hutchinson.

Sapey, B., Spandler, H., & Anderson, J. (2015) Introduction. In: Spandler, H., Anderson, J. & Sapey, B. (eds.) *Madness, distress, and the politics of disablement*. Bristol, Policy, pp.1–9.

Schlick, M. (1939) *Problems of ethics*, trans. Rynin, D. New York, Prentice-Hall. Available from: https://archive.org/stream/problemsofethics029364mbp/problemsofethics029364mbp_djvu.txt [Accessed 10 November 2016].

Smail, D. (2005) *Power, interest, and psychology: The elements of a social materialist understanding of distress*. Ross-on-Wye, PCCS Books.

Spandler, H. (2014) Letting madness breathe? Critical challenges facing mental health social work today. In: Weinstein, J. (ed.) *Mental health: Critical and radical debates in social work*. Bristol, Policy Press, pp.29–38.

Spandler, H. & Anderson, J. (2015) Unreasonable adjustments? Applying disability policy to madness and distress. In: Spandler, H., Anderson, J. & Sapey, B. (eds.) *Madness, distress, and the politics of disablement*. Bristol, Policy, pp.13–25.

Tavistock and Portman NHS Foundation Trust (2017) Meeting the challenge, making a difference: Working effectively to support people with personality disorders in the community. Available from: http://repository.tavistockandportman.ac.uk/864/1/Heather_Wood_-_MeetingTheChallenge.pdf [Accessed 14 November 2017].

The Guardian (2015) Austerity and a malign benefits regime are profoundly damaging mental health. Letter, 17 April. Available from: https://www.theguardian.com/society/2015/apr/17/austerity-and-a-malign-benefits-regime-are-profoundly-damaging-mental-health [Accessed 10 May 2017].

Thoits, P. A. (1985) Self-labelling processes in mental illness: The role of emotional deviance. *American Journal of Sociology*. 91(2), pp.221–249.

Twinley, R. (2014) Mental disorder. In: Taylor, P., Corteen, K. & Morley, S. (eds.) *A companion to criminal justice, mental health and risk*. Bristol, Policy Press, pp.165–166.

UK Government (2007) *Mental Health Act 2007*. Available from: www.legislation.gov.uk/ukpga/2007/12/contents [Accessed 10 May 2017].

UK Government (2005) *Mental Capacity Act 2005*. Available from: https://www.legislation.gov.uk/ukpga/2005/9/contents [Accessed 27 November 2017].

Weinstein, J. (ed.) (2014) *Mental health: Critical and radical debates in social work* (series eds. Ferguson, I. & Lavalette, M.). Bristol, Policy.

WHO (2001) *The world health report 2001. Mental health: New understanding, new hope*. Geneva, WHO.

6

MEDICALISATION

Resistance or replacement?

The idea that woes can be explained, classified, and treated as if they were malfunctions of the body or mind has been resisted since the Classical period, and was parodied in a Greek play (see Chapter 3). In the last two centuries, resistance has been motivated by people's experience of coercive methods of treatment that draw their rationale from the illness myth. Most of the worst excesses of measures to contain or treat people judged to be mentally ill have been curbed. This applies to the institutionalisation of thousands of people in asylums or hospitals and to aggressive physical methods of 'treatment'. However, through its widespread acceptance by the public, the concept of mental illness has a more subtle and pervasive influence, in which medicine and psychiatry play a merely supportive role. In fact, members of these professions have often been the strongest critics of medicalisation. The main question addressed in this chapter is whether the practices that grow out of a concept of mental illness can be refined, moderated, and effectively 'improved', or whether entirely new ways of explaining and tackling woes are needed. New approaches are, in fact, already waiting in the wings (see Chapter 8). In this chapter, I review ways in which medicalisation has been resisted, and whether attempts to make the concept of mental illness more acceptable have been successful.

Resistance from the 'mentally ill', their carers, and other advocates

Active resistance to involuntary treatment and physical methods began as far back as the eighteenth century (Porter, 1987; Chamberlin, 1990; Campbell, 2009; *The mental health history timeline*, MHHT, n.d.). The key players in this story were usually individuals who had been admitted involuntarily to an institution or they, or their carers, were distressed by the 'treatment' they had received. Resistance has led to the formation of political pressure groups and to the development of alternative services outside the mainstream. One letter to *The Times* newspaper in 1970 led to the formation of the National Schizophrenia Fellowship, which later became the charity Rethink Mental Illness. The letter writer, John Pringle, the parent of a young man diagnosed with schizophrenia, seemed neither opposed to nor in favour of the concept of mental illness. He wrote almost entirely about what could be done in a practical way to change an inadequate system of care and rehabilitation. His suggestion was to abandon mental hospitals and set up 'small residential settlements where their [i.e. patients'] basic needs, including protection from impossible stress, can be provided in a mutually supportive environment' (Pringle, 1970). In the United States, Judi Chamberlin (1978) campaigned for alternatives to conventional psychiatry, having experienced inpatient treatment herself.

People who have been motivated by their experiences to bring about change have described themselves as 'survivors', 'ex-service users', or 'psychiatrised persons'. Campbell sums up their main beliefs as follows:

> . . . belief in the essential competence of people with a mental illness diagnosis; belief in the value of self-help and collective action; belief in the possibility of self-organisation by service-users and survivors; belief that people with a mental illness diagnosis may have special expertise to offer society as a result of their personal experience.
>
> *Campbell, 1999: 199*

Service-users/survivors could be described as engaging in identity politics in the sense that their campaigning is linked to an identity that stems from an oppressive experience (Pilgrim, 2005). They aim to raise public awareness and bring about a radical change of attitude towards an oppressed group. This almost certainly entails replacing disrespectful descriptive labels with a form of language chosen by the group. It also means that even small expressions of a discriminatory attitude are deemed unacceptable. However, service-users are not united by a shared rejection of the concept of mental illness nor by how they think their problems should be dealt with.

Some campaigners simply wish to improve services for the 'mentally ill', and they accept mental illness as a valid description of a personal state of affairs. Charities advocating on behalf of the so-called mentally ill are concerned about the way society discriminates against a person with a psychiatric diagnosis. They do not see it as part of their function to offer a radical critique of the status quo. Resistance and reform have therefore been promoted under different banners. Two important issues are, first, on whose behalf resistance is being promoted and, second, how the group that resists prefers to be labelled.

Naming a movement

Morrison (2005: 161) refers to persistent debate over the right to decide what words to use to identify the movement, its membership, and how an individual relates to psychiatry. Resistance takes many forms, with different factions often taking diametrically opposed views. The problem of naming would not exist, or would exist in an entirely different form, if the mythical status of mental illness were to be acknowledged. The concept of mental illness gathers in an extremely diverse set of woes and so there is little to be gained by choosing a replacement concept with a similarly global remit. Slade (2009b: 5) states that he will use the term 'mental illness' to describe the experience itself. As a concept is not something that is experienced, he must mean experiences that are interpreted to signify mental illness. Slade is critical of a medical framework, but his phenomenological strategy for wriggling out of it does not work when medical terminology continues to be used. Slade refers to 'consumers' but this can only mean a consumer of a medical service: 'Developing a sense of agency can be a painful process for the consumer, often starting with accepting that they have an illness' (Slade, 2009b: 167).

Political activism feeds off a sense that it is necessary 'to face up to things together'. People who have had a bad experience of the way their problem or crisis has been dealt with often feel rejected or alienated. They may benefit from talking to others who have had similar experiences. As the banner of mental illness covers a multitude of different woes, resistance has tended to coalesce around specific targets of discrimination, where the sense of sharing the same issues is obvious. When community initiatives with a broad remit have been undertaken, there is a tendency to form smaller sub-groups that have a narrower objective (e.g. Holmes, 2010). Moreover, with the advent of the Internet, it is now far easier for people with similar woes to group together for concerted action. Consequently, there is little need for an overarching label that encompasses all forms of 'distress' or 'woefulness'.

The identity of being a survivor makes sense when bad experiences are seared in a person's memory. It implies surviving psychiatric care and, most probably, episodes of extreme distress. However, there is something paradoxical about a movement that is opposed to current mental health practices whose members define themselves in a way that can only reaffirm the concept around which the services they received were organised. In effect, it can be equivalent to declaring 'I am or have been mentally ill.' Chamberlin (1990), in her account of the history of the 'ex-patients movement', remarks that for the more radical members, any discussion that included mental health terminology was considered suspect. These members were united by a sense of unjustified discrimination and oppression, and any diagnosis they may have received was unimportant.

As a campaigning identity, 'ex-user' or 'survivor' has the disadvantage of excluding people with similar experiences who have not been processed by the mental health system. Moreover, many people who have been diagnosed as mentally ill at one time or another, and have received psychiatric treatment, may no longer see this experience as contributing to their current identity but are nevertheless motivated to campaign on behalf of those who do. Although abolition of the concept of mental illness would not eliminate prejudice, discrimination, or the need for coercive controls in some instances, it should prove possible to create new non-illness identities that refer to a type of problem or difficulty in a more neutral way. In any case, some earlier categories of disorder, such as homosexuality, have already been de-medicalised. What was abhorred in one historical period ceases to be noteworthy in another.

Abolition of a global concept of mental illness should eventually lead to a withering away of stereotypic images of so-called mentally ill people. Discrimination against people who are distressed by their own behaviour or who distress others cannot, however, be expected to disappear. There seems to be an irrepressible tendency to judge other people and find some of their beliefs or characteristics abhorrent; despised out-groups are constantly being formed. Some people would still be described as 'a bit funny in the head', 'having one screw missing', or 'impossible to deal with'. In other words, there will always be a need to foster tolerance of differences between people. The pejorative phrases just listed are not automatically associated with a loss of respect and they do not necessarily represent an attack on personhood and human rights. They are examples of intolerance rather than medicalisation.

Prevalent fantasies of madness can be a major source of anxiety in people who interpret relatively minor anomalies in their behaviour as a sign of their impending disintegration and mental collapse. There is little doubt that the very word 'mental illness' can conjure up fear. Our collective memory includes terrifying images of straitjackets, shackles, and brain surgery. Sayce, who has lobbied on behalf of people discriminated against on grounds of mental illness, describes how as a teenager she experienced episodes of intense anxiety and an eating problem related to a feeling that she was too fat: 'The truth was that I was terrified of losing control, of being "mad", and could only cope by pushing away attempts at help from parents and friends' (2000: 8).

Sayce did not enter psychiatric treatment, and her reluctance to do so may have been due to her 'fear of what it might mean to be "mentally ill"' (ibid.: 9). The arguments in her book oscillate between wanting to see a new language emerge, linked with greater tolerance, and wanting people 'to drop discriminatory attitudes towards people diagnosed as mentally ill' (ibid.: 12).

Within the survivor movement there is a group of people who celebrate their own 'madness' (Curtis et al., 2000). Madness is not a psychiatric diagnosis and therefore does not imply medicalisation. The problem with an approach that celebrates madness as 'difference' is that the term is as elastic as the concept of mental illness. Do we, for instance, celebrate the eccentricity of the hoarder who fills their home with precious junk? Whatever we might think, the person's partner might not view it in the same way, and if the hoarder lives in an apartment block, there might be objections from other residents about fire hazards and attracting vermin. One example of changing perceptions of 'difference' is the UK Paedophile Information Exchange, founded in 1974, which existed as an organisation lobbying for a change in the age of consent. It received some government funding and was briefly affiliated with the National Campaign for Civil Liberties. It was officially disbanded in 1984, and is unthinkable as an organisation in 2017.

The point of citing these examples is to suggest that any departure from what is considered acceptable or tolerable varies so much that it is impossible to celebrate 'difference' per se. There has been some accommodation to the removal of medical labels in so far as the term 'service-user' has replaced 'patient' in the UK National Health Service. However, in an obviously medical context, the connotation of 'patient' or 'service-user' is likely to remain the same. As Pilgrim (2005) notes, who is it that is being served when the service is not one that is wanted? New labels have a habit of retaining the same meaning as the older politically incorrect terms they replace.

Some psychiatrists have accommodated to resistance by working collaboratively with service-users (see below). There has also been a move to re-label mental illness as a disability or impairment, presumably with the intention of de-stigmatising mental illness, encouraging tolerance, and paving the way for social provisions that recognise 'difference'. However, anything short of abolishing the concept of mental illness gives the present mental health system an opportunity to accommodate to and absorb new terminology (Boyle, 2013). As Chamberlain (1990) argues, it is not enough for groups 'to speak for' consumers of mental health services. She asserts that a basic liberation principle is for people to speak for themselves. In her view, the survivor movement faces formidable obstacles because the concept of mental illness is a part of everyone's vocabulary.

Modes of resistance

Chamberlin (1978) emphasises the importance of consciousness-raising in order to dispel confusion about the 'whys' of woes. She believes that people who have been labelled (or label themselves) in ways that undermine their self-worth and power can benefit from understanding their predicament from entirely new perspectives. Resistance to medicalisation usually begins with a declaration to create a new vocabulary. For instance, organisations set up alongside statutory services (and not necessarily in competition with them) insist on their own names for the people who use them: the Leeds Survivor Led Crisis Service refers to their 'visitors' and 'callers' (Venner and Noads, 2013).

Chamberlin (1978: 86) sets out three distinct models for promoting alternatives to the mental health system. In the partnership model (not one that she favours herself), professionals and non-professionals work together. Chamberlin believes that in spite of the participants being partners, it is unavoidable that a clear demarcation persists between those who give and receive help. This model is viewed as an alternative in name only. In the supportive model, membership is open to all people, but professionals are excluded except when performing an indirect role. In the separatist model, the service is open only to users or ex-users of the psychiatric system. Anyone else is seen as interfering with the task of consciousness-raising. Members support each other and run services themselves.

According to Chamberlin, partnership models usually degenerate into a service run by professionals or administrators, who are likely to endorse a mental illness ideology. This is an understandable concern if relinquishing the concept of mental illness requires a radical transformation of perspective. Furthermore, resistance to established authority is often very difficult for people who have suffered historically from physical, emotional, or sexual abuse. Campaigners always stress the need to foster 'empowerment' and 'social justice' because this relates directly to the experiences of their members. For people who are accustomed to being disempowered, taking control of their lives and feeling justified in doing so contributes in a major way to a resolution of the effects of their abuse. Chamberlin therefore argues for the exclusion of professionals not simply because they can hinder consciousness-raising but because she feels it is necessary for people to learn to exercise power themselves. Ex-users of services can share their experiences and have them validated by peers who fully understand the meaning of what is being communicated. Group members can challenge each other with empathy and have their opinion respected. Those who initiate and organise services outside the mainstream system are usually ex-users who feel that they have passed successfully through a healing process and believe that they can help others to do the same. Chamberlin is concerned that the word 'empowerment' has been absorbed into political rhetoric and is in danger of losing any meaning. She counters this danger by listing what an empowerment process means in practice, which she breaks down into 15 components (Chamberlin, 1997).

An interesting example of inadvertent consciousness-raising and empowerment is described by McKeown, Cresswell, and Spandler (2014). A trade union representing workers in a social services department in Sheffield, England, enlisted the support of a local organisation for survivors of the mental health system. The survivors entered and occupied empty social service premises, supported by striking workers. On return to work seven months later, the workers found that some survivors began to question their actual need for services:

> Survivors, having tasted power and freedom through political activism, were no longer content to revert to the role of a passive recipient of welfare predicated, as such a role unquestionably is, upon a distinction between them being labelled as 'mad' and us (the workers) being legitimized as 'mentally healthy'.
>
> *McKeown, Cresswell, and Spandler, 2014: 156*

This example reinforces the view that partnership models could be a disservice to the people they purport to help. Beresford and Menzies advocate the development of partnerships, seeing them as a form of collaboration that opposes present psychiatric practices. For these authors, 'service user/survivor' is a useful political identity (2014: 78). They distinguish between two types of partnership, one 'consumerist' and the other 'democratic'. In the former, the service-user is consulted for their feedback and is offered limited choice, whereas with a 'democratic model' the user has more say in how a service is run. The authors argue for an alliance between professionals, researchers, and service users, in which the latter are equal partners.

Burstow (2014) is sceptical that change can be brought about from within. She believes that the mental health industry is so powerful that strategies for changing the present system must be carefully worked out in a slow process of attrition. More recently, she argues that psychiatry must simply be dismantled because any form of resistance is met by accommodation and absorption (Burstow, 2015: 21). Burstow describes one example of accommodation that generated heated discussion within her own organisation (ibid.: 44). This concerned whether to endorse a New York bill banning involuntary electroshock treatment for children under age 16. On the one hand, endorsement could be seen as lending legitimacy to electroshock under some circumstances (which was in conflict with the organisation's aim of complete abolition), but on the other hand, abolition for the under-16s was at least an advance in the right direction. (This was the position that was eventually adopted.)

There exist many examples of a democratic model in which the interests of researchers and survivors do coincide. Academics who contribute to the discipline of 'mad studies' are opposed to 'sanism', a term that refers to all forms of oppression of the mad. The intention is to convey the message that all kinds of difference should be celebrated. However, 'identification with difference' is probably a minority position within the group of people who currently seek help from mental health services.

Beresford and Menzies (2014) quote the sentiments of David Oaks, former director of MindFreedom International, when he called for a 'non-violent revolution' (Oaks, 2008). Oaks was speaking at a conference on Madness, Citizenship and Social Justice. Despite 32 years as an activist, Oaks sent out the rather dispiriting message that over this period the biomedical approach had increased its hold over mental health services and was spreading its tentacles to the developing world. He called for more protests and greater activism, even though, based on his own experience, it would seem that the message has not been getting through. He preceded his call for a non-violent revolution with the remark that 'mild reform is a trap'.

Oaks wanted to see changes to current services, especially government support for non-drug alternatives to the problems of so-called mental illness: 'There ought to be a full range of voluntary, humane, safe options and alternatives offered to all those who choose to use them, including mutual support, jobs, housing, peer-run programs, nutrition, advocacy, quality counseling, and wholistic approaches' (Oaks, 2008: 13).

This is not so different from Sedgwick's call, 25 years ago, for alternatives to institutionalised care based on a non-medical concept of asylum (Sedgwick, 1982). He argued for the provision of crisis centres, supervised group living, and a 'campus' of community homes for ex-psychiatric patients. However, Sedgwick did not see this as a revolution in mental health ideology but simply an argument for greater investment by the State in social welfare. As he stated: 'There should be little doubt that, for radicals and reformers within the politics of mental health, "working within the system" means working within the publicly funded system of health and social welfare provision' (ibid.: 244). Sedgwick believed that reformers and revolutionaries who turned to 'alternative sectors' or care outside the public-welfare system condemned themselves to 'marginality' and 'irrealism'.

Investment in mental health services (at least in the UK) has been begrudging, and it is the alternative sector that has grown in size and influence. In an effort to spend wisely, governments call for practice to be based on 'best evidence', but the research feeding into this exercise typically employs psychiatric criteria for problem definition and therapeutic outcome (Hallam, 2013). The State is wedded to the concept of 'mental health/mental illness', which narrows its vision and restricts the kind of service it is willing to fund. Sedgwick cannot be criticised for saying that there is an important role for the State but he, too, adhered to a conventional view of mental illness. He believed in 'real need' and 'specialised care', and disparaged alternative therapy 'as a loose label covering virtually any kind of chat about even the most transient and everyday problem or conflict' (Sedgwick, 1982: 223). He dismissed radical manifestoes of the later 1960s and 1970s for being extraordinarily ambitious and unrealistic. One 'unrealistic' manifesto he quoted called for 'giving the individual an awareness of the personal and social conditions that provoked his crisis' and creating 'denormalising, de-psychiatrising, joyous actions and passions, and work-relationships which completely change the function of work into an intense, un-alienated activity of struggle towards social change' (ibid.: 238).

These aims seem less idealistic today than they must have done 25 years ago. Nevertheless, Sedgwick (ibid.: 195) did acknowledge the validity of self-help and radical alternatives to institutional psychiatry (Cresswell and Spandler, 2009). He supported the demands of the Mental Patients Union (MPU) in London in 1973 when they protested against coercive measures, physical treatments, poor information, lack of access to case-notes, and poor aftercare, amongst other deficiencies (Sedgwick, 1982: 228). However, he noted that the MPU and similar movements lacked ideas about what was needed to replace existing practices.

Beresford and Menzies (2014) point to 'new discourses' being developed by mental health service users/survivors, and they predict that the future will see unprecedented change resulting from collective action. They argue that academics and professionals should hitch themselves to this movement. It is possible that professionals will, in future, make a significant contribution (direct or indirect) to 'supportive' and 'separatist' models in Chamberlin's terms. So much research has been undertaken on ways to conceptualise and overcome common problems in living that its contribution is unlikely to be ignored. Voluntary organisations endorse much of the self-help literature written by professionals (or generate their own), and enter into supportive or partnership relationships with professionals.

Nevertheless, Oaks' warning that 'mild reform is a trap' is ominous. For instance, in commenting on the organisation SANE, a mental health charity that is committed to the concept of mental illness, Beresford and Menzies (2014: 94) observe that public fears of mental illness had been generated by the case of a service-user's unprovoked murder of a bystander on a railway platform. They conclude that a problem arising in these kinds of cases is the unavailability of psychiatric help when a service-user has sought it out. This begs the question whether there might be an alternative to the way that people with homicidal impulses are detected and monitored, perhaps offering sanctuary where possible, thereby avoiding the deplorable consequences of a senseless murder. New discourses imply new solutions, and not a fall-back on the tried and tested model when the public is perceived to be at risk.

Service-user involvement in mental health services

In light of the extremely low status of institutionalised patients of sixty years ago, it is welcome that service-users can now contribute to the development of mental health policy, to research, and to the promotion of alternative forms of support outside mainstream services. They can rightly claim to refer to themselves as 'experts by experience'. It is, however, a certain kind of expertise and one that needs to be supplemented by other traditions. Beresford (2013: 193) states that 'there aren't as yet survivor controlled conceptualisations of madness and distress' but this remark seems to imply that knowledge could (or should) belong exclusively to the group who acquires it. It is not clear what the control of knowledge by service-users would mean in this context.

A recent report published in collaboration with the UK National Service Users Network (NSUN), based on research financed by the Department of Health, gives a detailed account of the involvement of service-users in the mental health system (Faulkner et al., 2015). It very carefully avoids any challenge to the concept of mental illness apart from quoting statements from service-users. 'They talked of the need to avoid language felt to be stigmatising by certain groups of people, for example, "mental illness", or (for some people) "drug user"' (ibid.: 38).

It is quite clear that the term 'service-user' in the NSUN report refers to people who are expected to be long-term dependents on the system or in intermittent need of inpatient care. There is also a strong emphasis on the needs of people who act as carers. However, it is not helpful to lump together all people who use the mental health system as if they fall into a group that needs enduring support. Even within this group, service-users may share little in common. The position of someone who views their crisis as a temporary one and is treated with respect by the mental health service, differs from a service-user who is dependent on various forms of enduring support or feels under threat of being legally detained and treated involuntarily. The former are more likely to be described as having a 'mental health problem' whereas the latter are 'mentally ill'. The authors of the NSUN report are very much aware that service-users are supplicants:

> Genuine co-production would mean a culture shift in services; if service-users are to be equal partners in the commissioning of services, they would also need to share in the responsibility and accountability for those services. Some of the service-users consulted for the report did not feel that this was realistic. Equally, some were pessimistic about the potential for clinicians and commissioners to share their power sufficiently to allow for service-users to make a difference.
>
> *Faulkner et al., 2015: 36*

Service-users have been employed as advisers in management, research, and policy making. One study found that the experience of taking on these positions (for the service-users) only reinforced their inferior status and did not remove the perception that they were mentally ill (Lewis, 2015).

In support of a partnership model, Beresford and Menzies (2014) cite the example of the project SURE (Service User Research Enterprise) (SURE, n.d.), situated in an academic department with associated inpatient facilities for people diagnosed with severe mental illnesses. Service-users are involved in the design, execution, and dissemination of research investigations into topics such as a consumer perspective on ECT, the acceptability and experience of inpatient care, the evaluation of health and social care interventions, the measurement of the side effects of neuroleptic drugs, and tailoring pharmacological treatments to a person or group's biological make-up. The nature of these research questions does not inspire confidence that there is any departure from current practices, and they do not illustrate 'the struggle against biogenetic psychiatry' which Beresford and Menzies aim to advance (2014: 89).

Critical psychiatry

Critical psychiatry is how psychiatrists currently working within the profession, but also critical of it, prefer to describe their stance (Critical Psychiatry, n.d.). Moncrieff and Middleton (2015) go to the heart of the matter when they state that '100 years of research has failed to produce evidence of any defect in the structure or function of the brain, or any other part of the body, that is specific to schizophrenia' (2015: 2). Schizophrenia is the so-called mental illness for which a biological explanation seems most credible, given that the behaviour associated with it is difficult to comprehend and often equates with madness in the public imagination. It may give rise to a perceived need for coercive control. In the absence of a medical rationale, Moncrieff and Middleton believe that: 'The social control of unwanted behaviour would have to be openly and democratically debated, rather than hidden away behind the language of medicine and "treatment"' (ibid.: 4).

The dilemma for critical psychiatrists is how they can criticise the biomedical model yet continue to justify their position as medical specialists wielding considerable power. A serious critique of the concept of mental illness implies letting go of the linguistic, professional, legal, and ideological frameworks in which it is embedded. For many critical psychiatrists, the message has to be watered down. Bracken calls for 'a primary focus on meanings, values and relationships' but 'this is not to deny that psychiatry should be a branch of medicine' (2014: 242). He wants to overturn a scientific/determinist/technological mindset but this is not about 'demonizing drugs or biological psychiatry' (Bracken, n.d.). Double writes that: 'The mechanisms by which mental illness emerges in an individual are psychologically mediated' (2005: 57). If so, it is a puzzle why the phenomenon that 'emerges' is called an illness. Some internal critiques are weaker still. Charland is opposed to the medicalisation of woes, especially the commercial exploitation of fictional illnesses, but his gripe is 'no ideological or political romantic threnody in defense of a utopia without medical terms and concepts' (2013: 162). Charland seems to believe that psychiatry could only be replaced in a utopia, presumably because he cannot imagine any other way of responding to people's problems and suffering.

Bracken and Thomas (2009) see a way forward through the concept of recovery and an alliance with service-users, many of whom reject the medical model. Service-users are seen as the 'experts' when it comes to the fundamentals of what is at stake. They are experts in one sense but they are still required to collaborate with the 'acknowledged experts' in a relationship of unequal power. In any case, service-users' expertise is in large measure acquired through having to cope with a managerially engineered system of services that they have been obliged to use.

Mental illness as impairment or disability

Some critics of medicalisation have turned to concepts of impairment and disability as a way of normalising the behaviour of the so-called mentally ill. These concepts have the effect of changing social expectations so that what was formerly discrediting is brought within a wider compass of 'normal', and adjustments are made, if necessary, to make this possible. According to the 2006 United Nations Convention on the Rights of Persons with Disabilities, a disability can be 'psychosocial' in nature. Any legislation that includes disability as a criterion (as mental health law obviously does) is held to be discriminatory (Gordon and O'Brien, 2014). The political and legislative implications of treating so-called mental illness as a disability or impairment have not yet been worked out. I will limit myself to examining the rationale of this kind of re-labelling.

One rather obvious motive is that 'it', however the impairment is conceived, is given a non-pejorative label, which opens up the possibility of granting rights to welfare under the umbrella of disability. Cook and Jonikas (2002) state that:

> . . . recipients would be viewed as having a right to voluntary, recovery-oriented services and supports, as well as personal assistants, job and education coaches, and full access to information technology that would allow them to learn about and advocate for their rights while offering and receiving peer support.
>
> *Cook and Jonikas, 2002: 327*

One powerful objection to this approach is the difficulty of defining what the psychosocial disability is without resorting to the language of illness or disorder. Cook and Jonikas refer to psychiatric disability as if it were obvious what this meant. At times they imply that this means people diagnosed with a psychiatric disorder but this could apply to around one-quarter of the population. When they state that: 'It is also critical that they be permitted the liberty to determine their own actions according to personally-developed goals' (2002: 317), this can only refer to people whose rights have already been taken away on grounds of mental illness. The way forward is surely to abolish the concept of mental illness rather than re-label it as a disability. A problem or woe can be disabling but in many cases the reason is obvious and need not be attributed to a 'disorder' in the person.

The disability route leads to a labyrinth of difficult issues relating to diagnosis, social identity, and tortuous policy-making (see the collection of chapters in Spandler, Anderson, and Sapey, 2015). One of the contributors to this book draws a comparison between the 'psycho-emotional disablism' suffered by disabled people with the same sort of name-calling, stigma, and abuse directed at people diagnosed with a mental illness (Reeve, 2015). It is true that calling someone a nutter or a cripple are equally abusive. Reeve is aware of the difficulty of attaching a concept of impairment/disability to so-called mental illness but proceeds on the basis that it can be done. Reeve deals with the problem of psychiatric terminology by preferring to use the term 'mental distress'. This raises the potential size of the group of impaired and disabled people in the population to close to 100 per cent. In any case, 'mental distress' is double-talk because, from other allusions that Reeve makes, it is a euphemism for people who are described as having a severe mental illness. Reeve argues that what people who are 'different' actually want is acceptance, rather than social inclusion on grounds of a psychiatric diagnosis and associated impairment/disability. This is true but, as noted earlier, it is acceptance per se, not acceptance despite carrying any form of label. In practice, any newly minted term for the 'mentally impaired' is destined to become an innocent-sounding version of 'nutter'.

Reeve's main argument is that mental distress feels like impairment. It cannot be disputed that so-called mental illness can feel like illness. The substantive issue is whether the assumed underlying bodily dysfunctions/impairments actually exist, and assuming that they were demonstrable, what could be done to respond to them. In the absence of this knowledge, Reeve simply accepts 'mental distress as a valid way of being' (2015: 110). However, most people do not want to be distressed, which is not to say that they cannot be distressed for valid reasons. A person may wrongly believe that their distressing experiences are invalid in the sense that they should not be having them. A common therapeutic strategy is to validate the reality of the causes of distress with the ultimate purpose of reducing distress. It is also possible to validate an experience of distress by encouraging a person to accept, own, and embrace it (e.g. grief, disappointment, justified anger). In this case, it is still assumed that accepting the experience is a transitional stage towards an overall reduction of distress.

Beresford (2016: 320) argues that new ways of delivering welfare support, such as direct payment schemes, challenge the distinctions and divisions between those reliant on welfare and those who are not. With 'user-controlled support', a person can think more creatively about how they might want to enhance their well-being. Designed mainly for people with a disability, the idea has been extended to service-users, now seen as being impaired/disabled. Although this system gives the service-user a greater say, they must account for all the money they spend as required by local government auditing departments. Consequently, this distinguishes them from ordinary consumers. The scheme is aimed chiefly at people who have been described as having 'serious mental illness', an important group, but it links the concept of service-user with an enduring identity of impairment. People who are both on welfare and considered to be mentally ill are in fact a small minority compared to the size of the population liable to be given a diagnosis of mental illness at some time in their life.

Beresford (2015) is in favour of finding a way to link disability studies with the mental health user/survivor movement but mainly on grounds of shared concerns, giving added political weight. He dissociates himself from a definition of a mental health problem in medical terms and sees unifying possibilities in the neurodiversity movement and in 'mad' studies. Neurodiversity is a concept developed by people given diagnoses such as autism and dyslexia who regard their condition as an expression of human diversity, a neurotype rather than a neuropathology (Graby, 2015). A somewhat similar position is taken by the hearing voices movement, which rejects the way that a 'symptom' that is not necessarily distressing has been pathologised. Voices are assumed to have meaning, and, in any case, exist on a continuum with everyday experience. In so far as there are neural correlates for all forms of behaviour, we are all neurotypes, and the implications of neurodiversity are similar to those of abolishing the concept of mental illness.

A risk of making people who are both diagnosed as mentally ill and also dependent on welfare the primary focus of resistance to medicalisation is that this tactic detracts attention from the much wider employment of the biomedical model to people who certainly would not see themselves as impaired or disabled. In his own experience of being a service-user, Beresford states that the psychiatric and drug treatment he received left him confused and disorientated. It was only later 'that a skilled and supportive psychologist put me on the road to regaining control' (2013: 189). The key word here is 'control'. Recovery, for Beresford, meant a lack of dependence on others (i.e. statutory services). One connotation of the label 'disabled user' is that he or she is never really expected to be fully in control.

Beresford's second possibility for an emergent identity is madness. Mad studies began in the Mad Pride movement of the 1990s and developed into an academic discipline that draws upon the literature and experiences of people diagnosed as mentally ill. It supports the position of people who are happy to regard themselves as 'mad'. According to Beresford, 'mad studies' has the potential to be a unifying political focus and new banner for a variety of interest groups, and he believes that it will engender different social understandings and strategies (ibid.: 258).

One such vision of madness has taken inspiration from R. D. Laing's writings in the 1960s. Farber re-defines the whole debate in spiritual terms. In brief, madness is for him a non-rational altered state of consciousness (ASC), a derangement in a spiritual process that everyone has to go through in order to remain sane. An ASC is said to be bad if it leads to insanity but it can also be good as a potentially valuable experience that is spiritually regenerative. For Farber, insanity is not a psychiatric term; 'normal' people can be insane as can whole societies if what they are doing has the potential to destroy human survival. Farber's theory is that 'the mad constitute a vanguard in the effort to bring change to an insane world' (2012: 9). Although many of Farber's speculations seem far-fetched, they have the merit of drawing attention to processes that are appropriately described as spiritual growth. They also prompt a search for meaning in ASCs.

Community-based clinical practice

Practices based on the concept of mental illness can be resisted by slowly transforming them into something guided by concepts of community, ecology, and system. Lightburn and Sessions contrast ineffective traditional clinical practice with 'community-based clinical practice' (2006: 23). This is a partnership model that has the mental health of the whole community in its sights. It emphasises continuity of support rather than short-term crisis-led interventions for individuals with 'mental illness'. The aim is 'to avoid institutional care' (ibid.: 29) and 'build capacity in support of the mentally ill and their families' (ibid.: 32).

The weakness and strength of this type of partnership model is that the ideas of agencies on the ground can outrun the philosophy of their funders. On the one hand, departure from customary practice may diminish a funder's willingness to endorse them wholeheartedly (or at all). Mental health policy is not necessarily based on rational considerations; decisions may reflect a change of political ideology or follow from service reorganisation and budgetary cutbacks. On the other hand, innovation at the professional coalface has the potential to be taken up politically and change policies and funding decisions. Demonstrations of what can be done well can serve as a model even if the funding is short term and a project has to end prematurely (e.g. Dore, Feldman, and Gelles, 2006).

It is a tall order to get community-based practices right when an individual, her or his family, the larger community, and statutory authorities have conflicting objectives. For instance, problems have arisen in community-based integrated family centres:

> . . . While family centers are friendly, open door places, where parents can walk in without referrals and be welcomed to join in center programs, they are also places that engage in protective work with parents who are mandated to receive help because their children are at risk for abuse or neglect.
>
> *Warren-Adamson and Lightburn, 2006: 262*

The recovery model

The belief that a person can recover from a mental illness implies that illness exists. In other words, in a medical context, recovery implies previous illness. (One can, of course, recover from other woes in a different sense.) Slade (2009b), in a major review and a guide to services based on the concept of recovery, refers on the first page of his book to a person 'struck down by mental illness'. Diseases can strike a person down but woes more often *grind* one down. A person who 'recovers' might believe that they were once 'ill' or believe, instead, that they were never ill because their original problem had been misidentified. The term 'recovery' is usually employed by psychiatrists to mean that a person learns how to mitigate the impact of symptoms of an illness that is ongoing. Another meaning of recovery that Pilgrim and McCranie (2013) extract from the recovery literature is the idea of a meaningful journey that is unique to the individual. In a metaphorical sense, life itself is an illness from which we all suffer, and for which we have to find a personal answer. To continue the analogy, the so-called mentally ill are not in a separate hospital ward signposted 'risk of contagion, keep out'; everyone is liable to infection and admission. However, to use illness in this analogical way implies that we have some notion of what illness means literally. We cannot speak logically of de-medicalisation when every type of illness is figurative.

A philosophy of recovery could be interpreted as a form of resistance to medicalisation when it counters the belief, stemming from early psychiatric texts, that so-called severe mental illness is a chronic condition with a very poor prognosis. This view of schizophrenia as a chronic deteriorating illness from which there is no recovery or cure has now changed in the light of later empirical studies (Bellack, 2006; Warner, 2010). The recovery model does not pull back from a biomedical concept of illness but it does cease to regard people as patients in passive receipt of treatments that aim for a cure (Shean, 2010). In sum, it treats people as struggling human beings with a capacity for change like anyone else. The metaphor of treatment is exchanged for education, support, help, re-skilling, sharing, etc. In some programmes there has been a strong focus on empowerment and personal meaning (e.g. Deegan, 2005). In fact, the concept of recovery is said to have grown out of service-users' experience of what was helpful to them based on their own experience. Recovery has now become a very influential concept within mental health services but often remains anchored in the assumption that those in need of services must recover from an underlying disorder, e.g. alcohol or opioid abuse or schizophrenia (Anthony, 1993).

The concept of recovery retains the medical metaphor when it is taken to mean a reduction of symptoms. For Warner (2010), recovery is a clinical strategy to help a person struggling with a severe mental illness. Typically, professionals collaborate with service-user organisations that operate independently of the mainstream service. Warner thinks implicitly in terms of medical outcomes by referring to the proportion of seriously mentally ill people who achieve 'complete recovery' or 'social recovery'. He writes at length about the role of a person's insight into the nature of their illness, so it is unclear whether the severely mentally ill can ever return to being 'normal'. They are the walking wounded however well they do. A medical perspective on recovery can also be discerned in research into therapy for 'common mental disorders'. In randomised control trials, outcome measures have been divided into 'disorder specific' and 'non-disorder specific' (e.g. Baardseth et al., 2013). The former are measures of symptoms and the latter are assessments of general well-being in areas such as work, relationships, and social activities.

In the absence of a concept of mental illness, recovery, at least in a medical sense, would lose any meaning. Abolition would have to be accompanied by a radical reframing of the social response to problematic or deviant conduct. Rather surprisingly, Slade, who initially referred to people being struck down by mental illness, ends his book with the following sentence: 'The recovery agenda will be complete when there are simply groups and communities and networks in which there is no caseload because there is no service – there are only people' (2009b: 236).

If this statement is meant seriously, the recovery movement is a Trojan horse that will eventually bring about de-medicalisation.

The concept of recovery has been criticised from a social justice perspective: 'Simultaneously, Western states are downloading their social responsibilities to the voluntary sector and to citizens themselves' (Howell and Voronka, 2012: 1). The concern is that responsibility is devolved to the citizen who is invited to show resilience and create a 'meaningful life' despite illness. However, given widespread dissatisfaction with statutory services for the so-called mentally ill, this 'downloading' would not be unwelcome if it could be achieved without an endorsement of medicalisation and proved popular. State funding would still be needed to provide resources for individuals, groups, communities, and voluntary-sector organisations that took on responsibility for dealing with particular woes. However, if a health rationale were to be removed, Howell and Voronka might be right to suppose that the State would find few reasons to aid the woeful to any degree at all.

McDermott (2014) warns that a recovery philosophy risks ignoring the political and social context in which so-called mental illness arises. The concept of recovery can be sidetracked into an agenda of assigning responsibility to the individual and ultimately providing a justification for the withdrawal of services. When there is a drive 'to get people independent and off benefits', support might be withdrawn once this has been achieved, ignoring the fact that continuing support is often needed. The problem is compounded by having high local authority eligibility criteria for support. The Catch 22 is that support leading to recovery is withdrawn when it is actually needed to sustain recovery. A service driven only by 'crises' is one way to reduce costs but early and sustained efforts may in the long run be more cost-effective.

Diagnosis as a moral verdict

Szasz (1970) compared psychiatric diagnostic practices with inquisitorial methods to ascertain whether or not a person was a witch. Officials representing church dogma were appointed in order to determine whether a person was colluding with the enemies of orthodox religion (i.e. with the devil). Szasz viewed the power invested in these officials as similar to the powers of psychiatrists to designate some people as 'legally' ill. Sarbin and Mancuso (1980: 100) follow Szasz in treating the diagnosis of schizophrenia as a moral verdict. Just as witchcraft was a cultural phenomenon tied to a mythology of spiritual forces, so mental illness is assumed to be a mythology dependent on occult causes and widely held beliefs in its existence. Some witches accepted that they really were witches and some mentally ill people believe that they really are ill. Sarbin and Mancuso (ibid.: 103) cite evidence (Manis, Houts, and Blake, 1963) that those who enter hospital begin to adopt the terminology of mental illness while those who remain the longest do not. One interpretation of this finding is that acceptance of the ideology is evidence of cure. Sarbin and Mancuso comment that this is not so different from the inquisitor's judgment that the confessing witch was 'saved but burned'.

How then do psychiatric patients understand the purpose of 'treatment' and its relationship to their atypical experiences? Do they expect the State to take responsibility for their condition? Interviews with several people given a diagnosis of psychosis and receiving psychological therapy revealed a rather confusing mixture of perspectives (Messari and Hallam, 2003). The interviewees had no doubt that their experiences were 'real', just as, no doubt, a witch is entirely convinced that people are surrounded by dark forces. However, they tended to oscillate between viewing their experiences as a truthful rendition of reality to seeing them as a symptom of illness. Psychological therapy was construed in several, partially incompatible, ways: as educational, as healing, as a kind of friendship, and as compliance with the aims of the psychiatric institution. It seems that the interviewees could construe their 'treatment' as helpful and coercive at the same time. The study raises questions about the meaning of an open and honest dialogue when, in the background, psychiatric and therapeutic imperatives are subtly concealed.

The argument that diagnosis is a moral verdict rather than the ascertainment of a medical condition leads to a situation in which society has to confront, more directly, the moral grounds for providing welfare. The seemingly default position that a person is responsible for taking care of their own destiny has to be matched by a recognition that the State has a responsibility to respect human rights and to ensure that conditions are in place to make a worthwhile life possible. According to Harper and Speed (2012), policy documents such as the Department of Health's *No health without mental health* (DOH, 2011) and Rethink's *100 ways to support recovery* (Slade, 2009a) get the balance wrong: 'Rather than effecting social change, the marginalized other is required to change their personal outlook' (Harper and Speed, 2012: 12). Harper (2010) points out that many of the demands of the Mental Patients Union (MPU) set up in 1972 have not yet been met, especially those concerning collective social justice, such as the abolition of irreversible physical treatments, compulsion and seclusion, and right to treatment of choice.

Any new proposal to change mental health policy would have to take into account discrimination against people who contravene social norms and also public fears about the behaviour of 'mad people'. New policies would be faced by at least three tasks: (1) countering marginalisation (i.e. through acceptance, empathy, trust, re-establishing a sense of personhood and entitlement to human rights) (2) rectifying woeful circumstances (e.g. unemployment, lack of adequate housing, social support, or child care, problems of debt, etc.) (3) resolving specific woes (e.g. family conflict, low mood, self-harm, lack of interpersonal skills, fears, addictions, compulsive habits, etc.). In the future, the field of mental health is likely to fragment into distinct areas of personal and social concern, each with its own preferred resolution. In fact, this has already begun to happen. The concept of mental illness appears to be a hindrance rather than a help to future thinking.

Summary

The distressing and sometimes traumatic experience of hospitalisation for mental illness has led to the publication of a large number of survivor narratives and the formation of grass-roots resistance movements. They embody a wide range of opinion, from acceptance to complete rejection of the concept of mental illness. Grass-roots organisations may operate independently or in various degrees of partnership with professionals. A number of psychiatrists are highly critical of some of their own professional practices and have allied themselves with the survivor movement. There are also attempts to normalise so-called mental illness by redefining it as impairment or disability. Mental health services have adapted to criticism by changing their terminology and by working in the community on a more democratic basis. The recovery movement aims to promote a good quality of life for service users rather than focus on the treatment of 'symptoms'. The long history of resistance to the medicalisation of woes, its diverse manifestations, and the possibilities opened up by grass-roots alternatives, pose challenging questions for current mental health policy. These have not yet been satisfactorily answered.

References

Anthony, W. A. (1993) Recovery from mental illness: The guiding vision of the mental health service system in the 1990s. *Psychosocial Rehabilitation Journal*. 16(4), pp.11–23.

Baardseth, T. P. et al. (2013) Cognitive-behavioral therapy versus other therapies: Redux. *Clinical Psychology Review*. 33, pp.395–405.

Bellack, A. S. (2006) Scientific and consumer models of recovery in schizophrenia: Concordance, contrasts, and implications. *Schizophrenia Bulletin*. 32(3), pp.432–442.

Beresford, P. (2016) *All our welfare: Towards participatory social policy*. Bristol, Policy Press.

Beresford, P. (2015) Distress and disability: Not you, not me, but us? In: Spandler, H., Anderson, J. & Sapey, B. (eds.) *Madness, distress, and the politics of disablement*. Bristol, Policy Press. pp.245–260.

Beresford, P. (2013) Experiential knowledge and the reconception of madness. In: Coles, S., Keenan, S. & Diamond, B. (eds.) *Madness contested: Power and practice*. Ross-on-Wye, PCCS Books, pp.181–196.

Beresford, P. & Menzies, R. (2014) Developing partnerships to resist psychiatry within academia. In: Burstow, B., LeFrançois, B. & Diamond, S. (eds.) *Psychiatry disrupted: Theorizing resistance and crafting the (r)evolution*. Montreal, McGill-Queen's University Press, pp.77–95.

Beresford, P., Perring, R., Nettle, M. & Wallcraft, J. (2016) *From mental illness to a social model of madness and distress*. Published by Shaping Our Lives. Available from: www.shapingourlives.org.uk/wp-content/uploads/2016/05/FROM-MENTAL-ILLNESS-PDF-2.pdf [Accessed 10 March 2017].

Boyle, M. (2013) The persistence of medicalisation: Is the presentation of alternatives part of the problem? In: Coles, S., Keenan, S. & Diamond, B. (eds.) *Madness contested: Power and practice*. Ross-on-Wye, PCCS Books, pp.3–22.

Bracken, P. (n.d.) *Beyond paradigms: Promoting a recovery agenda in mental health*. Available from: www.soteria.freeuk.com/Brackenbeyond.htm [Accessed 28 November 2017].

Bracken, P. (2014) Toward a hermeneutic shift in psychiatry. *World Psychiatry*. 13(3), pp.241–243.

Bracken, P. & Thomas, P. (2009) Beyond consultation: The challenge of working with user/survivor and carer groups. *Psychiatric Bulletin*. 33, pp.241–243.

Burstow, B. (2015) *Psychiatry and the business of madness: An ethical and epistemological accounting*. New York, Palgrave Macmillan.

Burstow, B. (2014) The withering of psychiatry: An attrition model for antipsychiatry. In: Burstow, B., LeFrançois, B. & Diamond, S. (eds.) *Psychiatry disrupted: Theorizing resistance and crafting the revolution*. Montreal, McGill-Queen's University Press, pp.34–51.

Campbell, P. (2009) The service user/survivor movement. In: Reynolds, J., Muston, R., Heller, T., Leach, J., McCormick, M., Wallcraft, J. & Walsh, M. (eds.) *Mental health still matters*. Basingstoke, Palgrave Macmillan, pp.46–52.

Campbell, P. (1999) The service user/survivor movement. In: Newnes, C., Holmes, G. & Dunn, C. (eds.) *This is madness; A critical look at psychiatry and the future of mental health services*. Ross-on-Wye, PCCS Books, pp.195–209.

Chamberlin, J. (1997) A working definition of empowerment. *Psychiatric Rehabilitation Journal*. 20(4), pp.43–46.

Chamberlin, J. (1990) The ex-patients' movement: Where we've been and where we're going. *Journal of Mind and Behavior*. 11(3), pp.323–336.

Chamberlin, J. (1978) *On our own: Patient controlled alternatives to the mental health system*. New York, Hawthorn Books.

Charland, F. C. (2013) Why psychiatry should fear medicalisation. In Fulford, K. W. M., Davies, M., Gipps, R. G. T. et al. (eds.) *The Oxford handbook for the philosophy of psychiatry*. Oxford: Oxford University Press, pp.159–175.

Cook, J. A. & Jonikas, J. A. (2002) Self-determination among mental health consumers/survivors: Using lessons from the past to guide the future. *Journal of Disability Policy Studies*. 13(2), pp.87–95.

Cresswell, M. & Spandler, H. (2009) Psychopolitics: Peter Sedgwick's legacy for the politics of mental health. *Social Theory & Health*. 7(2), pp.129–147.

Critical Psychiatry (n.d.) Available from: www.criticalpsychiatry.co.uk [Accessed 10 March 2017].

Curtis, T., Dellar, R., Leslie, E. & Watson, B. (2000) *Mad pride: A celebration of mad culture*. London, Spare Change Books.

Deegan, P. E. (2005) The importance of personal medicine: A qualitative study of resilience in people with psychiatric disabilities. *Scandinavian Journal of Public Health*. 33(66), pp.29–35.

DOH (2011) *No health without mental health: A cross-governmental outcomes strategy for people of all ages*. London: HMSO.

Dore, M. M., Feldman, N., and Gelles, A. W. (2006) Family of friends: Creating a supportive day care community to prevent child abuse and neglect. In: Lightburn, A. and Sessions, P. (eds.) *Handbook of community-based clinical practice*. Oxford: Oxford University Press, pp. 245–260.

Double, D. (2005) Beyond biomedical models: A perspective from critical psychiatry. In: Tew, J. (ed.) *Social perspectives in mental health*. London, Jessica Kingsley, pp.53–70.

Farber, S. (2012) *The spiritual gift of madness: The failure of psychiatry and the rise of the mad pride movement*. Rochester, VT, Inner Traditions.

Faulkner, A. et al. (2015) *Involvement for influence*, 4Pi National Involvement Standards. Available from: www.nsun.org.uk/about-us/our-work/national-involvement-partnership/ [Accessed 10 May 2017].

Gordon, S. & O'Brien, A. (2014) New Zealand's mental health legislation needs reform to avoid discrimination. *The New Zealand Medical Journal*. 127(1403). Available from: https://www.nzma.org.nz/journal/read-the-journal/all-issues [Accessed 10 May 2017].

Graby, S. (2015) Neurodiversity: Bridging the gap between the disabled people's movement and the mental health system survivors' movement? In: Spandler, H., Anderson, J. & Sapey, B. (eds.) *Madness, distress, and the politics of disablement*. Bristol, Policy Press, pp.231–244.

Hallam, R. S. (2013) *Individual case formulation*. Oxford, Academic Press.

Harper, D. (2010) Tensions and dilemmas in clinical psychology's relationship with the service user movement. *Clinical Psychology Forum*. 209, pp.35–38.

Harper, D. & Speed, E. (2012) Uncovering recovery: The resistible rise of recovery and resilience. *Studies in Social Justice*. 6, pp.9–25.

Holmes, G. (2010) *Psychology in the real world; Community-based groupwork*. Ross-on-Wye, PCCS Books.

Howell, A. & Voronka, J. (2012) Introduction: The politics of resilience and recovery in mental health care. *Studies in Social Justice*. 6(1), pp.1–7.

Lewis, L. (2015) Recognition politics as a human rights perspective on service users' experiences of involvement in mental health services, In: Staddon, P. (ed.) *Mental health service users in research*. Bristol, Policy Press. pp.87–104.

Lightburn, A. & Sessions, P. (2006) Community-based clinical practice: Re-creating the culture of care. In: Lightburn, A. & Sessions P. (eds.) *Handbook of community based clinical practice*. New York, Oxford University Press, pp.19–35.

Manis, M., Houts, P. S. & Blake, J. B. (1963) Beliefs about mental illness as a function of psychiatric status and psychiatric hospitalization. *Journal of Abnormal and Social Psychology*. 67, pp.226–233.

McDermott, D. (2014) The problem with recovery, In: Weinstein, J. (ed.) *Mental health: Critical and radical debates in social work*. Bristol, Policy Press, pp.63–70.

McKeown, M., Cresswell, M. & Spandler, H. (2014) Deeply engaged relationships: alliances between mental health workers and psychiatric survivors in the UK. In: Burstow, B., Diamond, S. and LeFrançois, B. (eds.) *Psychiatry disrupted: Theorizing resistance and crafting the revolution*. Montreal, McGill Queen's University Press.

Messari, S. & Hallam, R. (2003) CBT for psychosis: A qualitative analysis of clients' experiences. *British Journal of Clinical Psychology*. 42, pp.171–188.

MHHT (n.d.) The mental health history time line. Available from: http://studymore.org.uk/mhhtim.htm#TheEarlyYears [Accessed 10 November 2016].

Moncrieff, J. & Middleton, H. (2015) Schizophrenia: A critical psychiatry perspective. *Current Opinion*. 28, pp.1–5.

Morrison, L. J. (2005) *Talking back to psychiatry: The psychiatric consumer/survivor/ex-patient movement*. New York, Routledge.

Oaks, D. W. (2008) Prospects for a nonviolent revolution in the mental health system during a time of psychiatric globalization or how we so-called lunatics may help save your mad planet! Lecture given at 'Madness, citizenship and social justice: A human rights conference', Simon Fraser University, 12 June. Available from: www.mindfreedom.org/who-we-are/david-w-oaks/madness-citizenship.pdf [Accessed on 10 March 2017].

Pilgrim, D. (2005) Protest and co-option: The recent fate of the psychiatric patient's voice. In: Bell, A. & Lindley, P. (eds.) *Beyond the water towers: The unfinished revolution in mental health services 1985–2005*. London, The Sainsbury Centre for Mental Health.

Pilgrim, D. & McCrainie, A. (2013) *Recovery and mental health: A critical sociological account*. Basingstoke, Palgrave.

Porter, R. (1987) *Mind forg'd manacles: Madness and psychiatry in England from the Restoration to Regency*. London, Athlone.

Pringle, J. (1970) Letter to *The Times*, 9 May. Available from: https://www.rethink.org/about-us/people-and-history/john-pringles-letter [Accessed 10 December 2017].

Reeve, D. (2015) Psycho-emotional disablism in the lives of people experiencing mental distress. In: Spandler, H., Anderson, J. & Sapey, B. (eds.) *Madness, distress, and the politics of disablement*. Bristol, Policy Press, pp.99–112.

Sarbin, T. R. & Mancuso, J. C. (1980) *Schizophrenia: Medical diagnosis or moral verdict?* Oxford, Pergamon.

Sayce, L. (2000) *From psychiatric patient to citizen: Overcoming discrimination and social exclusion*. Basingstoke, Macmillan.

Sedgwick, P. (1982) *Psycho politics*. London, Pluto Press.

Shean, G. D. (2010) *Recovery from schizophrenia: Evidence based theories and practices*. Cairo, Hindawi Press.

Slade, M. (2009a) *100 ways to support recovery: A guide for mental health professionals*, Rethink recovery series (Vol. 1). London, Rethink.

Slade, M. (2009b) *Personal recovery and mental illness: A guide for mental health professionals*. Cambridge, Cambridge University Press.

Spandler, H., Anderson, J. & Sapey, B. (eds.) (2015) *Madness, distress, and the politics of disablement*. Bristol, Policy Press, pp.99–112.

SURE (n.d.) Service User Research Enterprise. Available from: www.kcl.ac.uk/ioppn/depts/hspr/research/ciemh/sure/index.aspx [Accessed 10 November 2016].

Szasz, T. (1970) *The manufacture of madness: A comparative study of the Inquisition and the mental health movement*. Syracuse, NY: Syracuse University Press.

Venner, F. and Noad, M. (2013) A beacon of hope: Alternative approaches to crisis – learning from Leeds Survivor Led Crisis Service. In: Coles, S., Keenan, S., and Diamond, B. (eds.) *Madness contested: Power and practice*. Ross-on-Wye, PCCS Books, pp.332–348.

Warner, R. (2010) Does the scientific evidence support the recovery model? *The Psychiatrist*. 34, pp.3–5.

Warren-Adamson, C. and Lightburn, A. (2006) Developing a community-based model for integrated family center practice. In: Lightburn, A. and Sessions, P. (eds.) *Handbook of community-based clinical practice*. Oxford: Oxford University Press, pp.261–284.

7

WELL-BEING AND MENTAL HEALTH

I have argued in earlier chapters that 'mental health' is an over-inclusive concept that is used in a slippery and inconsistent fashion. Well-being is another concept that can take on different meanings. It can refer to a momentary feeling state (happy, satisfied, etc.) or to a person's reflection on their life as a whole – how meaningful and fulfilling it seems to be. My preference for using the words 'woe' and 'woefulness' is not because they are more precise. I intend them to cover a broad range of circumstances, both personal and social in origin, that may share little in common apart from being undesirable. The circumstances they refer to can imply a loss of well-being in any of its senses. Each person's life is unique, and this may explain why it is difficult to define woes and well-being in a way that could apply to everyone. Perhaps for this reason, researchers have resorted to simple scales of satisfaction or happiness to cover all possibilities.

Without knowing the basis upon which a person completes a scale measuring well-being, its usefulness as a guide for social policy is limited. It seems preferable to focus on more clearly defined specific woes in their social context. When placed in context, the meaning of a woe can be negotiated with the woeful individual, increasing the chance of showing it to be potentially temporary, situational, and solvable. In so far as a number of people share the same kind of woe for similar reasons, the broader social policy implications should become apparent.

Research into the links between mental health and well-being has not been conducted by studying specific woes in context. Instead, researchers have examined the relationship between measures of so-called psychiatric disorder and scores on simple scales of well-being removed from any social context. The most widely held view at present seems to be that there are degrees of being 'mentally ill' and degrees of enjoying a state of 'well-being'. This perspective on the matter follows logically from the idea that so-called mental illness (like physical illness) has three separate components, namely, underlying disorder/disease, signs and symptoms that reflect the presence of disorder/disease, and the personal and social effects of being disordered. The latter typically amount to a loss of well-being in various forms. For instance, an 'anxiety disorder' is defined psychiatrically by its 'symptoms', which have a knock-on effect on well-being, such as avoiding activities that would normally be useful or pleasurable. The analogy with physical illness is only approximate because in anxiety disorder, there is no underlying disease process, and the distinction between its 'symptoms' and their wider effects is arbitrary.

The research I review in this chapter is therefore flawed from the start, and few useful conclusions can be drawn from it. In any case, the terminology of mental illness differs fundamentally from that of well-being, leading to a mismatch between the methods of investigation that researchers employ. Consequently, it is difficult to relate the findings in each field.

Despite these intrinsic limitations, it is important to try to clarify what is meant by 'positive mental health' and how it relates to health in general. It is also relevant to review opinion within the emerging field of 'positive psychology', which has steered a path away from medicalisation onto topics such as resilience and happiness. Research conducted by positive psychologists has thrown some light on how people's woes and well-being are linked. It is also of interest to find out what people themselves understand to be the main sources of their well-being. Before reviewing research that helps to dispel some of the conceptual confusion, I will examine current assumptions that have helped to generate it.

Woes and a generic concept of health

As I have pointed out in earlier chapters, 'health' has been understood to have two main aspects: firstly, the presence of disorder or dysfunction, and secondly, a person's sense of 'well-being'. The promotion of well-being has been regarded as one of the functions of a health service. In the case of mental health, well-being takes precedence because disorder is rarely demonstrable. Of course, any so-called psychiatric disorder is bound up with a person's life circumstances. The 'symptoms' of 'mental illness' consist chiefly of behaviour that has an obviously negative effect on well-being. The severity of these effects depends on a person's individual circumstances. For example, the effects of severe insomnia (assuming this to be a disorder) are likely to vary according to whether a person is working, has young children to look after, can rely on social support, etc. A person's resources and their 'symptoms' (and vulnerabilities) are therefore intimately connected. This has led to the idea that well-being (positive mental health) prevents (or is a defence against) 'mental illness'. Health services have also promoted well-being on the assumption that this policy would yield economic benefits, such as reducing the need for health care.

According to the constitution of the World Health Organization, well-being is an integral component of physical and mental health. Health is 'a state of complete physical, mental and social well-being and not merely the absence of disease or infirmity' (WHO, n.d.).

The complete well-being of the individual is inconceivable without a benign social milieu in which the individual is able to function well. Therefore, according to the WHO's definition, the range of knowledge that is potentially relevant to health goes far beyond the scope of medical disciplines. The WHO definition could be seen as a territorial claim equivalent, say, to a definition of education that includes every possible form of learning. The idealism captured by the WHO's definition tends to fall short when it is applied in the field of mental health. Regardless of its claims, the WHO structures mental health policy in predominantly medical terms – that is, as the prevention and elimination of mental illnesses or disorders, not the fostering of well-being. The scope of medical knowledge is simply too narrow to do justice to the WHO's broad definition of health. Other disciplines have been co-opted but these have been described as, for instance, 'medical sociology' or 'professions ancillary to medicine', as if the medical aspect of health is the primary concern.

One WHO report is devoted to mental health promotion, where it is admitted that 'the activities of mental health promotion are mainly sociopolitical' (WHO, 2004: 26). Having identified what might be causing so-called mental illnesses, it remains an open question whether medical expertise would be needed to change the conditions that produce them. The UK Foresight Mental Capital and Wellbeing Project (Foresight, 2008) covers numerous topics, including employment, housing, urbanisation, exposure to crime, and debt. A clear exception where medical knowledge would be needed concerns developmental causal factors that have biomedical health implications (e.g. the pre-natal and peri-natal environment, genetic defects, diet, infectious diseases). Although developmental and medical factors of this nature have been linked to the later incidence of a variety of so-called mental illnesses, there are few examples of 'common mental disorders' (as they have been called) being associated in any specific way with risks of this kind.

As already noted, the WHO's efforts have been directed primarily towards curing or preventing illness and not towards fostering their wider conception of health. As Desjarlais and colleagues put it: 'Mental, behavioral, and social health problems are an increasing part of the health burden on all parts of the globe . . . hundreds of millions of women, men, and children suffer from mental illnesses' (Desjarlais et al., 1996: 4).

Mental illnesses are sometimes referred to as if they actually meant something as tangible as a heart attack. For instance, it has been claimed that:

> Mental illness accounted for more disability adjusted life years lost per year than any other health condition in the U.K. and the figures for 2004 show that 20% of the total burden of disease was attributable to mental illness (including suicide), compared with 16.2% for cardiovascular diseases and 15.6% for cancer.
>
> *Atlas of Variation in Healthcare, 2011*

Mental illness as a catch-all health condition is hardly meaningful. It could be argued with equal force that physical illness accounts for 80 per cent of the burden and mental illness only 20 per cent.

According to the Foresight report, 'an estimated 30% of GP consultations have an underlying mental-health cause, many of which have a socio-economic basis, e.g. debt, family breakdown, trauma, bullying at work, etc.' (2008: 22). The report states that many GPs do not currently feel it is their job to help patients seek support to address these social risk factors. Recent UK mental health policy still focuses on individual pathology rather than attempting to offer a community-wide service that deals with woeful circumstances (see Chapter 8).

The WHO has addressed its ideal conception of health by developing a broad-brush quality-of-life scale that covers many areas of well-being as well as some non-specific health indicators such as energy, discomfort, and quality of sleep (De Vries and Van Heck, 1997). The scale is intended to be used in the context of medical practice – that is, providing supplementary information for patient care, measuring change after treatment, improving doctor-patient relationships, evaluating health care, and monitoring the effects of changes in health policy. Although a measure of this kind has practical uses, it is hard to see it as a research tool that will elucidate the many causes of a less-than-ideal state of health. Moreover, the term 'mental ill-health' usually refers to psychiatrically defined conditions, not to a lack of well-being.

Attempts to define positive mental health

Jahoda (1958) offered an early analysis of the concept of positive mental health which is worth discussing in detail because it covered the essential issues. She drew upon writers who were having the greatest influence at the time, such as Abraham Maslow, Gordon Allport, Erich Fromm, Harry Stack Sullivan, and Erik Erikson. The source of their ideas was weighted towards adults who were functioning fairly well, a group that was probably receiving psychotherapy.

Jahoda's book was prompted by a concern of social decision makers to find ways of promoting a 'mentally healthy society'. Jahoda rejects the idea of defining positive mental health as the absence of mental illness because, apart from some rare exceptions, she thinks it impossible to draw a clear line between the 'ill' and the 'healthy'. She also rejects a definition in terms of behaviour that is statistically normal because she thinks there is no reason to suppose that the majority in a population are 'healthy' (Jahoda, 1958: 16). In any case, she argues that the choice of a reference group, and the selection of which characteristics to measure, already presuppose a non-statistical concept of health. Nor does Jahoda see much merit in equating positive mental health with a feeling state of happiness, well-being, or satisfaction, pointing out that these concepts disregard the social context and/or the specific situation in which a person is located, which could be a morally unjust one.

The literature that Jahoda reviewed in 1958 makes frequent reference to 'the self', and a state of mental health was related to various constructions placed upon this complex concept. In one respect at least, introducing the concept of self raises the level of discussion beyond a simple notion of well-being as a feeling state. A self is an attribute of a person, and personhood is a social status that has a bearing on well-being. In order for social life to be possible at all (that is, for anyone to be considered a 'normal person'), it is necessary for that person to be a singular material entity, to conform to norms of honesty in social discourse, and to present a consistent narrative of their biography over time (Harré, 1998; Hallam, 2009: 55). There are limits on how many personal identities it is possible to enact in different circumstances, and in Western societies, there is a category for abnormal multiplicity (Hacking, 1995). In other words, there is pressure to display a consistent and integrated persona across all situations. While inconsistency is inevitable, when taken too far it may be considered 'sociopathic'. Jahoda notes that several writers emphasise a 'balanced self' or a 'unified outlook'. While disunity is generally seen as 'unhealthy', a certain amount of disunity can denote flexibility and resistance to stress. One objection to a concept of mental illness is that it tends to imply an unalterable and fixed pathology.

The self can be understood as a social construct – in effect, a virtual reality that acts rather like an interior imaginary person who is assessing, guiding, and planning in order to foster a persona that is acceptable to, and valued by, self and others (Hallam, 2009). For some people, this process clearly fails, and they may hold themselves in 'low self-esteem' or 'self-disgust'. There must be many reasons for a person to place a low value on their 'self'. For instance, enduring self-attributions may be influenced by internalised messages received from caregivers (e.g. being a worthless person), from gender, class, or racial stereotyping, or result from personal encounters with abusive individuals. Self-regarding attitudes are ways of construing reality, and when the attitude is negative, an illness interpretation is only one of the options available. To have a very negative opinion of self could be an illness to one person and a life challenge to another. The significance of a constructional perspective on self is that a person's self-report of their 'symptoms' or 'well being' cannot be taken at face value. The self-report measures employed to investigate health could be reports on illness states, a person's judgement on their circumstances, or tap into character traits that reflect how a person wants to present themselves to the world (Schwarz, 1999, and see below).

Based on her literature search, Jahoda (1958) identifies some of the key dimensions that have been assumed to compose a mentally healthy self. I have paraphrased them here and ordered them differently:

(1) A person accepts the limitations and possibilities of their situation. This implies an awareness of past actions, obligations, feelings, etc., and an anticipation of their continuing relevance in future.
(2) This awareness is not 'distorted', as judged by a reasonable observer. A person is willing to test their perception of reality for its correctness.
(3) There is an identity attaching to this awareness – i.e. it is integrated in the sense of providing continuity and consistency of meaning for self and others (see above).
(4) A person is able to satisfy their needs but also shows a capacity for adaptation and adjustment when required to do so.
(5) A person is motivated in the direction of growth or development – i.e. involved in new pursuits in order to expand their potential.

(6) A person is self-determining in the sense of following their own chosen standards and is capable of acting relatively independently of others.

Jahoda's analysis of positive mental health is consistent with the Aristotelian concept of *eudaimonia*, and is distinct from *hedonia* that refers to the quality of feeling states (Ryan and Deci, 2001). The principles she extracts are very general in nature and they do not rule out the possibility (or inevitability) of conflicting urges and moral dilemmas. In practice, the principles have to be reconciled with a person's philosophy, sense of spirituality, and their aesthetic, moral, and political values. Not all dilemmas can be resolved, and so, on these grounds, positive mental health is not always achievable. Negative feeling states such as depressed mood, anxiety, frustration, or discontentment can be interpreted, not as mental disorders, but as stages that are necessary in moving forward towards a more satisfactory (eudaimonic) form of self-expression.

Ryff and Singer elaborate their interpretation of a eudaimonic approach to well-being and summarise findings that relate to their Personal Wellbeing Scale. Their five principles are self-acceptance, positive relations with others, personal growth, purpose in life, and environmental mastery. Like Jahoda, their position is that well-being can only be understood with reference to a person (or their 'self') in a social context. For this reason, each assessment of well-being should take account of a person's individual and unique circumstances, and a standardised scale, though useful, can only approximate this ideal. Despite the methodological limitations of self-report, scores on their well-being scale have been found to correlate with physiological measures that indicate 'better neuroendocrine regulation, better immune function, lower cardiovascular risk, better sleep, and more adaptive neural circuitry' (Ryff and Singer, 2008: 32).

The identification of *principles* of well-being rather than *states* of well-being has advantages from a social policy perspective because they can be applied flexibly to different circumstances. An example is the 'Capabilities Approach' that emphasises a person's ability to act on behalf of what matters to him/her, taking account of their potential capability to make use of opportunities and the forms of valued being that are actually available to them (e.g. health, safety, education) (Sen, 1999; White, Imperiale, and Perera, 2016). This approach expands the scope of a concept of well-being by emphasising the need to explore systemic socioeconomic and political barriers that curtail a person's ability to achieve what they desire.

Jahoda argues that there are different ways to be 'mentally healthy' (1958: 66). Drawing upon an analogy with the false idea of an overarching theory of disease, she states: 'In the field of mental health, some believe that the dissolution of the "blanket concept" is the next strategic step' (ibid.: 68). If anything, quite the reverse has happened since she wrote these words. A biomedical concept of mental illness has become more entrenched, and well-being and life satisfaction have continued to be confounded with a need to treat or eradicate illness.

Measurement of well-being by means of self-report

Faced with the conceptual complexity of well-being and positive mental health, researchers have resorted to using operational definitions – that is, to concepts defined by the completion of an operation, such as answering a set of questions. This research strategy has been employed, for instance, in measuring intelligence, which has been defined as performance on a series of cognitive tests. When concepts are operationalised, researchers often (but need not) lose sight of processes that are theorised to underlie performance. These are referred to as latent variables or latent constructs. When measures of well-being are used to guide social policy, it is very important to understand what the underlying constructs are taken to be, and whether, in fact, the research evidence supports the assumptions made about them.

One widely used operational measure of well-being is the Warwick-Edinburgh Mental Well-being Scale (WEMWBS), which consists of 14 items asking about optimism, energy, feeling good, etc. (Tennant et al., 2007). The association between well-being and so-called mental illness is left implicit when the scale is explained to the public. As a UK National Health Service website states: 'Good mental wellbeing – some people call it happiness – is about more than avoiding mental health problems. It means feeling good and functioning well' (NHS, 2006). This statement is a good illustration of the difficulty in stating exactly what the scale is intended to measure.

A questionnaire with the related aim of assessing life satisfaction has been the subject of much research (Diener et al., 1985; Pavot and Diener, 2009). On Diener's questionnaire (The Satisfaction With Life Scale), the amount of agreement/disagreement with each of five statements is rated on a seven-point scale. The statements refer to whether life fulfils needs, is excellent, matches an ideal, etc. According to Pavot and Diener, scores on their scale are fairly stable (reliable) over short time intervals but much less so over longer periods, as one might expect if life satisfaction changes with circumstances. Ultimately, a life-satisfaction scale is whatever a respondent makes of it, and even if used consistently, it remains an unknown and idiosyncratic measure. An anxious or depressed mood might weigh heavily in one person's assessment of satisfaction but not at all in another's. As Pavot and Diener have commented: 'Until the cognitive processes involved in arriving at a life satisfaction judgment are known and understood, we will not fully know the meaning of high life satisfaction' (2009: 113). One quality-of-life questionnaire was found to correlate highly with a subjective measure of hope, and negatively with a measure of depression (Schrank et al., 2011), suggesting that a life-satisfaction score is related to a person's mood. If mood is one of the chief determinants of a person's response to a quality-of-life scale, the scale has limited value as a general-purpose indicator of life satisfaction.

Questionnaires to assess well-being, satisfaction, or quality of life are likely to be influenced by a person's character traits, such as a tendency to complain (to see the glass of life half-empty) or a tendency to give a socially desirable response, such as being grateful for being alive or wishing to be seen as 'coping'. These influences, known as response biases, could distort a statistical estimate of the actual relationship between a measure of so-called mental illness and well-being. In fact, distortion is very likely in the case of depressed mood. Kinderman and colleagues found that their own scale of well-being correlated highly with a measure of 'anxiety/ depression'. These researchers also assessed their respondents' 'response styles'. The results showed 'that ruminative response styles and self-critical causal attributions for negative events were associated with lower levels of wellbeing' (2011: 1042). They treat this finding as positive support for the validity of their scale but a less charitable interpretation is that well-being scores are to some degree a measure of personality characteristics such as 'whinging'. A low well-being score could be nothing more than an alternative indicator of low mood.

The relationship between well-being and so-called mental health

Keyes (2007) embraces an operational approach to measuring the relationship between 'mental illness' and 'positive mental health'. Westerhof and Keyes (2010) employed the Brief Symptom Inventory (BSI) (Derogatis, 1975) to measure mental illness. The BSI covers a wide range of distressing experiences (regarded as symptoms), which could be associated with all kinds of circumstances that are unrelated to a diagnosis of mental illness. The results of Keyes's research show that his self-report measures of mental illness and positive mental health (well-being) are somewhat independent of each other (Keyes, 2007). However, the two measures are negatively correlated (–.53), implying that they do share a considerable amount of variability in common. Given the existence of errors of measurement, response biases, and lack of clarity about the latent constructs the measures supposedly reflect, this style of research does not greatly advance our understanding. Worse still, it medicalises the language of positive mental health when Keyes refers to the 'symptoms' of positive mental health, its 'diagnosis', and its 'co-morbidities'.

Research with a similar aim was undertaken by Weich and colleagues, exploiting data collected from a random sample of the UK population in a survey designed to assess 'adult psychiatric morbidity'. From various questionnaires and interview schedules, they were able to extract items relating to well-being and showed that they could construct two scales from them that matched the concepts of *hedonia* and *eudaimonia*. Scores on these scales were related to various demographic characteristics as well as to a composite psychological symptom score derived from a clinical interview schedule. The symptom score was assumed to reflect the presence of common (non-psychotic) 'psychiatric disorders'. The authors' descriptive summary of their basic findings was as follows: 'The correlation between hedonic and eudaemonic well-being scores was +0.49. Correlations with CIS-R score [the symptom measure] were –0.61 for hedonic and –0.45 for eudaemonic well-being respectively' (2001: 25). The authors conclude that 'our findings demonstrate that wellbeing and mental disorder are correlated but independent dimensions' (ibid.: 26).

The claim of independence is unjustified because the authors selected well-being items on an a priori basis. In other words, their statistical analysis (principal components) did not analyse symptom items together with well-being items. It is therefore unknown whether common components could have been derived from the two types of item analysed together. 'Mental illness' is simply treated, de facto, as conceptually independent of well-being. Moreover, their conclusion seems incompatible with one of their stated assumptions about the meaning of mental health: 'We take "mental health" to mean the full spectrum of mental health states; "mental illness" refers to pathological disease states and "mental well-being" covers the positive end of the spectrum' (Weich et al., 2001: 24). The research they undertook presupposed independence of illness and well-being rather than a single spectrum of mental health.

In another UK study that separately measured psychological distress and well-being at age 33, the authors were able to make use of previously collected survey data on a cohort of live births in one week in 1958 who were followed from childhood through to adolescence (Hatch, Harvey, and Maughan, 2010). The participants were cross-categorised into two groups of distress and three of well-being (the latter, from 'languishing' to 'flourishing'). 'Pure distress' applied to 3.1 per cent of the sample and 'pure languishing' to 9.1 per cent. The authors found that 'the developmental profiles of these latter two groups were very similar (i.e. differences of +1/–1 percentage prevalence points) on factors such as oppositional or aggressive behaviour in childhood, as well as police contact and low aspirations upon leaving school in adolescence (ibid., 267). There were also similarities in social context, such as exposure to poor material conditions. The authors point out that they are not suggesting that the 'pure languishers' be medicalised' (ibid., 268). However, so many kinds of problematic conduct have been medicalised in recent decades that it is not clear why languishing deserves to be excluded. Reinterpreted as different kinds of woefulness, neither distress nor languishing need be medicalised.

Another developmental study related well-being scores on the WEMWB scale at age 60–64 to previously recorded information on the sample dating back to 1946 (Stafford et al., 2015).

The study did not focus on distress; rather, low well-being was related to childhood family circumstances. Father's level of care, mother's overprotection and neuroticism, and absence from school for childhood illness, were associated with lower levels of later well-being. It is very likely that these same factors would have predicted so-called mental illness had the latter been assessed. Presumably, they were not assessed on the untested assumption that well-being and so-called mental illness are distinct phenomena.

Positive psychology and 'mental illness'

Partly to counter a focus on the negative in medicalisation, a relatively new academic field has arisen called positive psychology (Ryan and Deci, 2001). It is argued that mental health research has underplayed people's resilience and similar positive qualities. Seligman, an active promoter of the positive psychology movement, has helped to shift the focus on to positive health. In his most recent account of well-being (which he calls 'flourishing'), he places less emphasis on a mood of happiness

(Seligman, 2002, 2011). His original conception proposed three components, namely the emotion/feeling of happiness, engagement in an absorbing activity ('flow'), and 'meaning'. He now defines 'the meaningful life' as 'belonging to and serving something that you believe is bigger than the self' (2011: 12). His concept of flourishing adds the elements of 'accomplishment' and 'positive relationships'. He argues that the five components he identifies can be treated as conceptually independent. Some components are tied to external referents, thereby removing the need to rely solely on subjective ratings of happiness or satisfaction.

In brief, Seligman argues that a focus on pathology has led to a neglect of well-being. He dates this trend to the late nineteenth century when 'we gave up character as an explanation of human misbehavior' (ibid.: 104). This, he believes, resulted in social sciences and psychology focusing on 'victims and negative emotions and alienation and pathology and tragedy' (ibid.: 105). Seligman believes that psychotherapy and drugs at best remove the disabling conditions of life (ibid.: 53). As he puts it: 'In general, talk therapy techniques all share the property of being difficult to do, no fun at all, and difficult to incorporate into your life' (ibid.: 48). In contrast, some of his positive psychology exercises are said to be 'fun'.

Most psychotherapists would agree with the emphasis that Seligman places on optimism and a positive attitude to life. However, in line with the common saying, 'no pain, no gain', it is likely that life will generally turn out to be a mixture of positivity and negativity. Woeful situations addressed by psychotherapists contain a mixture of what has been lost (some of which has to be given up forever) and what there is to gain (assuming this ambition to be realistic and attainable). The balance between positive and negative is likely to vary between individuals and types of woe. Seligman derides 'talk therapy' as being no fun, but people come to therapy because there are problems to be solved that obstruct their access to fun. The goals of therapy are never wholly framed in terms of the removal of woes because anything that solves a problem is likely to be viewed positively or it opens the gates to a positive state of affairs.

Nevertheless, positive psychologists are right to draw attention to the fact that academic disciplines concerned with mental health have been seduced by medicalisation and have accepted the construction of negative psychological states as illnesses and disorders. The more marginal traditions, such as humanism, existentialism, and phenomenology, have been more successful in sidestepping this trend. The influence of medicalisation seems to have grown over the past forty years despite opposition to it being axiomatic in early applications of a behavioural approach to therapy (e.g. Schwartz, Goldiamond and Howe, 1975). The concept of a 'behavioural repertoire' integrates the positive by taking all components of a person's behaviour into account when applying theory.

A fundamental criticism of positive psychology is that it does little to explain how problems and woes originate. Seligman is inclined to believe that negativity depends on a person's genetic endowment: 'It is likely that depression, anxiety, and anger come from heritable personality traits that can only be ameliorated, not wholly eliminated' (Seligman 2011: 52).

This is a counsel of despair rather than positivity and, in any case, does not match a lack of evidence for a genetic contribution for even some of the so-called major mental illnesses (see Chapter 4).

The results of Seligman's applications of positive psychology do not support his position that it is more important to address happiness and 'flourishing' than it is to relieve distress. For example, his school-based Penn Resilience Programme has been tried out in 22 UK schools for a large number of 11–12 year old children (Challen et al., 2010). The two-year follow-up evaluation was extended to a roughly equivalent group of children who did not receive the programme. The workshops themselves focused on negative thinking and social problem-solving skills, and followed manualised protocols.

The evaluation of the programme showed that it did not raise life satisfaction or behaviour scores but instead produced certain educational benefits and, for up to one year only, reduced scores on depression scales. The impact was much greater for more deprived and lower-attaining pupils and those who started the year with 'worse psychological health', particularly girls with these characteristics. This suggests that a focus on distress and deficits is not misplaced. According to pupils and facilitators, it was the social skills component (interpersonal skills around negotiation and assertiveness, and techniques for self-control) that was most commonly found useful. It was noted that the role of facilitator could be emotionally demanding due to the distressing nature of some of the real-life problems raised by pupils. The programme seems to have identified a need, and perhaps a gap, in the present curriculum, but not necessarily for the reasons envisaged by the programme designers.

Seligman's work with the US military focused on the negative inasmuch as it was designed to make soldiers more resilient to potentially traumatising experiences and to lower the incidence of 'post-traumatic stress disorder'. His military fitness training is based largely on cognitive therapy techniques that were developed by mental health professionals to help depressed or anxious people. The techniques focus on negative ways of thinking, and so they cannot fairly be described as an application of positive psychology.

Grenville-Cleave (2012), a positive psychologist, lists five barriers to well-being: 1. paying too much attention to negative emotions, experiences, and information; 2. neglecting to end experiences (when possible) on a high note; 3. comparing ourselves unfavourably with others; 4. adapting too quickly to positive events, and 5. being unable to control our impulses and channel our efforts. As general tendencies that apply to everyone, the first four barriers cannot easily explain the subset of people in a persistently woeful state who turn out to be amongst the damned rather than the elect. With regard to the fifth barrier to well-being, Grenville-Cleave cites Muraven and Baumeister (2000) as supporting the hypothesis that higher self-control is linked to higher well-being. This claim is debatable. Muraven and Baumeister compare a person's ability to exert self-control with a muscle that can be strengthened by regular exercise over the long term but is weakened by intense short-term use. For instance, they suggest that efforts to control excessive drinking, eating, or smoking may fail when a person experiences an external stress. The internal muscle is weak and a relapse occurs because a person's self-regulatory resources have already been used up. Difficulties in life are therefore attributed to a loss of 'willpower', an internal resource that involves conscious effort. Muraven and Baumeister (ibid.) assume that willpower gradually returns if a person has a rest period from further calls on a demand for self-control. They provide extensive experimental support for their model, although this is based on rather contrived laboratory tasks that may not mimic self-control in the real world.

Muraven and Baumeister state that 'self-control occurs when a person (or other organism) attempts to change the way he or she would otherwise think, feel, or behave' (2000: 247). They go on to state that 'Self-control is the exertion of control over the self by the self.' At first glance, it might seem safe to assume that people attempt to 'self-regulate' their woes. However, the resolution of a person's woe may have little to do with changing their own behaviour – rather, the objective could be to change someone else's behaviour or whatever is seen to be the cause of their woe. They may need to change ingrained habits to achieve these ends but this task need not be construed as a problem of self-control as Muraven and Baumeister conceive it. For instance, the 'self' that attempts to exert control over self may be the source of the problem. This self may have the misguided notion that greater self-control is the answer to its woe. For instance, most anxiety problems cannot be solved by willpower in the sense of exerting greater effort to control anxiety directly. The answer may lie in relinquishing control. Muraven and Baumeister describe self-control as an act that prevents or inhibits a dominant response (ibid.: 247) but relinquishing control (i.e. dis-inhibiting a controlling response) involves accepting a new definition of a problem or letting go of unhelpful (or unjustified) curbs on action. Being relieved of guilt does not, presumably, require an effort of self-control. While it may be true that accepting undeniable truths or giving up on a hopeless struggle are acts of sorts, these outcomes are usually forced on a person by circumstances or by insightful reflection.

There are certainly classes of woe for which it is credible to suppose that effortful control of a problematic situation consumes a resource with limited capacity. This accords with folk accounts of failure such as 'I just had no more to give' or 'I was hit by another whammy.' Nevertheless, willpower theories underplay all of the external resources that constitute props and supports for self-control. The latter are included under the concept of 'social capital' by other theorists (e.g. Orford, 2013: 163). Social capital has been defined in many ways but it refers essentially to the network of relationships in a community built on trust, shared resources, and ordinary wisdom. The advice of positive psychologists such as Seligman and Grenville-Cleave is, by contrast, centred on the individual: building character (e.g. becoming resilient) or changing attitudes, motivation, and mindset. While these personal attributes are important, there is a noticeable neglect of social capital in this literature, and also of the environmental conditions that help to foster the personality traits considered to be desirable.

A point in favour of positive psychology is that, as Seligman has stated, it reintroduces virtue into an approach to people's woes that had become medical and morally sterile. For him, well-being can be acquired through 'fun exercises' designed to train skills that foster virtuous behaviour. The usual meaning of a skill is that it is a means to an end, with the latter defining the value or virtue that exercising the skill is supposed to supply. In practice, skills do embody virtues. For example, training in assertiveness skills (Salter, 1949) has been linked to the United Nations Universal Declaration of Human Rights (Alberti and Emmons, 1974). The right to act assertively is justified by a claim to have a legitimate voice in a matter that is of direct personal concern. When teaching assertiveness skills, a therapist is often drawn into a moral debate about the pros and cons of, say, punishing a child for misbehaviour, holding an employer to account, or terminating contact with a family member. Like assertiveness training, the exercises and skills encouraged by positive psychologists have the intention of strengthening virtuous behaviour, thereby promoting a moral agenda.

The well-being exercises promoted by positive psychologists certainly make demands on a person's determination to live better and exercise choice. Echoing Thomas Szasz, Seligman states that 'responsibility and free will are necessary processes within positive psychology' (2011: 105). He does not think of this as a political statement but rather as pointing to essential 'causes'. However, Seligman does not give a causal account of free will or its failures. The reason that past theorists have focused so much on the negative aspects of life is the manifest inability of some people to exercise free will when they would very much like to do so. If we are not endowed with free will simply by virtue of being human, its development and strength need to be explained.

Well-being and social policy

Wood and Tarrier (2010) point out that a person's positive assets can predict negative states or buffer their impact (e.g. Johnson et al., 2011). They also stress the importance of positive well-being for its own sake. These views are reflected in recent changes to UK health policy that aim to promote well-being. Perhaps for this reason, a Public Health England survey of public attitudes in a random sample of UK adults was conducted with the purpose of examining the relationship between a person's well-being and whether or not they had received a diagnosis of mental illness (PHE, 2015). Approximately 25 per cent of respondents was currently experiencing or had had experience of a mental health problem. This sub-group was less likely to have a 'very high score' on a self-report scale of life satisfaction (20 per cent compared with 33 per cent of those without personal experience), indicating a modest association between the two measures. A majority of the respondents felt that they knew what to do to improve their own well-being but there were mixed views on the most important factors. The two most popular were relationships with family/friends and job/work-life balance. Other frequently chosen factors were the amount and quality of sleep, relaxing or having time out, and 'finances'. These findings, although of some interest, do not supply a ready explanation for an association between well-being and a diagnosis of mental illness.

The wording of the PHE report is confusing because the authors imply that well-being can be equated with being mentally healthy, a term that could mean either feeling well or not being afflicted by a mental disorder. They state: 'As we have seen, although a majority (72%) feel they *personally* know what to do to improve their mental well-being, only 36% agree that *most people* "know what to do to keep themselves mentally healthy"' (PHE, 2015: 5; original emphasis). The authors note that 70 per cent of respondents agreed that most people would 'know what to do to keep themselves physically healthy', double the proportion who would know how to keep themselves mentally healthy. It seems that for the public, mental health is a far more opaque concept than physical health.

There was one indication of an association between well-being and 'mental ill-health'. More people with personal experience of a mental health problem agreed that the things that affected their well-being were 'out of their control'. Similarly, a low life-satisfaction score was related to a (lack of) control over these things. The amount of perceived control was related to the level of social deprivation in the area in which a respondent resided, and this may have reflected, amongst other things, a lower income. In light of the outcome of the Penn Resilience Programme that the most deprived/depressed children benefited the most, the results of this survey also suggest that the greatest increment in well-being would be obtained by investing in the most socially disadvantaged segment of society (and their social circumstances).

Other surveys, such as those conducted by the Office for National Statistics, show that the strongest correlates of self-reported well-being are the state of a person's physical health, their employment status, and their relationship status (whether or not a person is in a marriage or partnership) (ONS, 2013). Consistent with these findings, a publication of the UK Department of Health states that 'improving subjective wellbeing is a worthy goal in its own right and can be instrumental to other outcomes – physical health, getting into work, and productivity' (DOH, 2014: 2). Although well-being is deemed to be worthy 'in its own right', the economic rationale for promoting it is also plain. The authors of the DOH document divide well-being into two dimensions: subjective and objective. The latent constructs that correspond to these dimensions are left unstated. Although the results of surveys (see above) indicate that there are objective determinants of well-being, it is not clear what is meant by an 'objective dimension' of well-being, if the latter is primarily a subjective appraisal.

In its arguments for promoting well-being, the DOH document notes that subjective well-being predicts increased life expectancy and survival in older populations, and can 'add 4–10 years to life' (2004: 9). This claim is supported by the results of a comprehensive review of the evidence (Chida and Steptoe, 2008), which concludes that well-being has positive effects on longevity in both healthy and diseased populations. This is an important and fascinating finding but until it is fully understood, it does not have clear policy implications. Correlation does not imply causation. Well-being may contribute to health through its association with other material factors. Moreover, it could hardly be denied that an awareness of illness and approaching mortality could to lead to lower ratings on a scale of well-being. The DOH document is slanted towards giving causal priority to subjective well-being. It is argued that 'compassion and kindness in hospitals' (2004: 2) could make a difference to health outcomes. However, kindness in hospitals is probably also a function of policies that determine nurse selection, training, and working conditions. It is further suggested that personal well-being 'influences the well-being and mental health of those close to us' (ibid.: 3), seeming to imply an obligation to stay cheery for others. The wording suggests that well-being can be distinguished from (but is allied to) mental health, which in this context presumably means 'mental disorders'.

The UK government has taken very seriously the proposal to focus efforts on indicators of well-being rather than relying too heavily on the monetary benefit of new policies. Layard (an economist) and Clark (a psychologist) argue that mental illness is 'probably the single largest cause of misery in Western societies' (Layard and Clark, 2014: 181). Buying into the disease model, the authors believe that there is insufficient spending on psychiatrists, psychologists, and therapists. This analysis has persuaded the UK government to make significant new investments in the provision of psychological therapy. This is welcome if it achieves its aims, but Layard links the initiative with population surveys of life satisfaction. In other words, it seems to be assumed that the causes of general well-being (life satisfaction) are similar to the causes of personal well-being. In reality, it is extremely difficult to draw causal inferences from a mass of correlations between different types of measure, e.g. objective indicators such as income and possession of luxury goods versus satisfaction with life in general versus day-to-day positive and negative feelings. The findings of a global survey of 132 countries revealed different predictors of satisfaction with life (a measure requiring a person to reflect generally on their circumstances) and the quality of their immediate experiences (i.e. positive or negative feelings) (Diener et al., 2010). These authors found that what they call 'social psychological well-being' (a concept akin to social capital) is very important for positive feelings. Consequently, conclusions drawn from a single measure of well-being or satisfaction are likely to be misleading.

Layard and other collaborators (A. Clark et al., in press) are struck by the fact that there has been little change in measured well-being in the UK over the past forty years, a finding replicated in other major advanced countries. Their preferred measure of well-being is based on a single question: 'Overall, how satisfied are you with your life, these days?' answered on a scale from 'extremely dissatisfied' (0) to 'extremely satisfied' (10). The lack of association between rising income and (flat) satisfaction levels is explained on the assumption that well-being is a relative measure. In other words, if subjective ratings are anchored by expectations shared with one's peers (or an equivalent comparison group), of what is 'good' and 'bad' in any given set of life circumstances, most people will fall between the two extremes and the average rating will remain constant. Clark and colleagues found that in several national data sets, the extent to which income predicts life satisfaction depends on an individual's income relative to that of others in their peer group as defined by age, gender, and region. They conclude that absolute income accounts for less than 2 per cent of the variance in life-satisfaction scores.

Layard and colleagues have investigated what it is that predicts life satisfaction over and above material circumstances, in order to provide pointers to the sort of policies that would enhance well-being for everyone. They see their task as explaining 'how all the different factors affect our life satisfaction, entering them all simultaneously in the same equation' (Clark et al., in press). This equation describes a fictional average person whose 'irrelevant attributes' have been removed by means of statistical adjustments. Clark and colleagues have drawn on data from large-scale surveys that have followed up respondents from childhood into adulthood. The findings for the fictional average are not uninteresting in themselves. The highest correlations for adults (even though they are of extremely small size) are obtained with (1) a measure of mental health (diagnosed depression/anxiety), (2) whether a person has a partner, and (3) the number of physical health conditions a person reports. With regard to a child's life satisfaction, the highest correlations are with the mother's mental health and the child's exposure to aggressive parenting. They conclude that from a social policy point of view, the cheapest way to make a difference to a nation's average life-satisfaction scores would be to treat more people for depression and anxiety. In fact, they phrase this suggestion as 'abolishing depression and anxiety'. They seem to assume that depression and anxiety are illnesses that can be cured, rather like a chest infection, ignoring all of the psychosocial correlates of these so-called illnesses (see Chapter 4).

As already pointed out, it is not easy to interpret scores on scales of self-reported well-being and life satisfaction. Layard and Clark adopt a hedonic definition of well-being as feeling good, and its opposite, feeling bad. They acknowledge that eudaimonic well-being, such as the ability to choose freely, to show compassion, and an inner life based on 'acceptance', all contribute to feeling happy. However, they are content with simple rating scales to measure feeling states of happiness or satisfaction, especially when averaged over the longer term (2014: 17). In their view, it is not possible to be both happy and unhappy at the same time (ibid.: 21), but, if so, it is difficult to know what to make of a person's average over time. If only instantaneous assessments are valid, any longer-term judgement of happiness is a different kind of appraisal that takes in many other aspects of life (as they seem to admit, ibid.: 33).

The economic argument for investing in psychological therapy is related to the assumption that people are rational maximisers who possess free will: 'From the various possibilities open to us, we choose whichever combination of activities will make us feel best' (ibid.: 26). Consequently, it is thought that people tend to err when they choose harmful short-term pleasures or fail to plan sensibly in the longer term: 'it is impossible to explain human action and human survival except by the desire to achieve good feelings' (ibid.: 26). On these grounds, the authors ought to attribute the recent rise (which they document) in alcohol abuse, clinical depression, drug addiction, youth suicide, and crime, to human irrationality. Instead, they point to our genes, poor upbringing, and family break-up. They cite as some of the empirically discovered correlates of self-rated happiness, the quality of family life, unemployment, trusted friends, physical health, political freedom, and personal values. If this is so, a simple subjective scale of happiness must cover up a wealth of complex interrelationships amongst social variables and material circumstances.

Despite this, Layard and Clark maintain that all the effective strategies for increasing happiness can be summed up in one message 'that we can liberate the positive force within us by dropping our negative self-perceptions and our inappropriate goals' (ibid.: 189). There is little evidence to support this belief. It stems from one brand of cognitive therapy whose actual mode of action is unknown and may, in fact, differ from its stated rationale (Hollon and DeRubeis, 2009; Watkins, 2009). Causal theories that focus on childhood experiences are dismissed as outdated, and they advocate cognitive and behavioural methods (CBT).

In practice, CBT (in common with many other forms of therapy) often focuses on the harmful consequences of an adverse childhood upbringing. The policy implications that derive from a focus on childhood would be programmes to support access to quality pre-natal and child care, comprehensive services for the prevention of child abuse, parenting skills, quality foster care, and related services (see Chapter 8). Instead, human woes are attributed to a person's attitudes (ibid.: 199), and schools are advised to teach as subjects 'the wisdom of the ages', not forgetting 'the causes and cures of illness, including mental illness, drugs and alcohol' (ibid.: 200). The importance of education cannot be underestimated, but this focus on knowledge and beliefs is far too narrow and focuses excessively on the individual.

If the argument is accepted that well-being is a relative measure, disadvantaged sub-groups (e.g. those disadvantaged materially or in terms of housing) will be less satisfied. A sub-group's anchoring (or reference) points are therefore influenced by objective conditions but it is departures from those conditions (better or worse) that are meaningfully related to variation in life satisfaction. For instance, gender gaps in income for doing the same job have generated dissatisfaction and led to strikes. The importance of the objective context is clear in a recent study of wage inequality and its relationship to the higher prevalence of 'depression' amongst women. In an analysis of a large US nationally representative survey of working adults, it was found that where female income was less than the matched male counterpart, the odds ratio for a so-called depressive disorder (i.e. the ratio of women to men) was significantly higher (Platt et al., 2016). Where female income was greater than the matched male, the higher odds ratio was significantly lower. To translate this finding into social policy, the choice seems to be between 'treating' women for 'depression' or legislating for income equality.

If a rating of well-being is a relative measure (i.e. judged in relation to a person's overall circumstances compared to peers), it should not be interpreted as a 'fixed quantity' similar to objective and material indicators of quality of life. A logical implication of its relative status would be to reduce social inequalities so that disparity between social groups was lessened. Policies to counter social adversities (and inequalities) such as inadequate housing, unemployment, physical ill-health, loneliness, etc., that are known to be related to subjective well-being, could well have a more beneficial influence on 'mental health problems' than making therapy services more readily available. Another consideration for policy makers is the fact that an individual's woes are often due to a combination of circumstances, many resting on accident, and these cannot be predicted and planned for. Consequently, the potential benefits of any social policy are intrinsically constrained by the effects of chance.

Summary

As currently conceived, mental health includes personal well-being, but current definitions of mental health are ambiguous and confusing. Services still focus on 'treatment' and 'pathology', with insufficient regard for the social context of woes. Research into positive mental health is mostly founded on self-report scales of happiness, satisfaction, or quality-of-life. It is argued that the methodology of this approach is weak and the measures themselves difficult to interpret. With regard to programmes to foster well-being, the positive psychology movement has inspired several initiatives. Their results only partially support the premises on which they are based, and positive psychologists are unable to provide a credible explanation for persistent and obdurate woes. Policies to enhance well-being have been promoted nationally for a variety of reasons (as an intrinsic good, as prevention of mental ill-health, and for their potential cost-saving benefits). It is suggested that the findings of well-being research are not yet sufficiently well understood to provide a sound basis for investing in individual therapy as a means of raising well-being for the population as a whole.

References

Alberti, R. E. & Emmons, M. L. (1974) *Your perfect right: A guide to assertive behavior.* Oakland, CA, Impact.

Atlas of Variation in Healthcare (2011) *Reducing unwarranted variation to increase value and improve quality.* NHS, November 2011. Available from: www.rightcare.nhs.uk [Accessed 10 March 2017].

Challen, A., Noden, P., West., A. & Machin, S. (2010) *UK Resilience programme evaluation; Final report.* Research Report DFE-RR097, London, Department for Education.

Chida, Y. & Steptoe, A. (2008) Positive psychological wellbeing and mortality: A quantitative review of prospective observational studies. *Psychosomatic Medicine.* 70, pp.741–756.

Clark, A., Fleche, S., Layard, R. et al. (in press) *Origins of happiness: Evidence and policy implications.* Available from: http://voxeu.org/article/origins-happiness [Accessed 10 May 2017].

Derogatis, L. R. (1975) *The Brief Symptom Inventory.* Baltimore, MD, Clinical Psychometric Research.

Desjarlais, R., Eisenberg, L., Good, B. & Kleinman, A. (1996) *World mental health: Problems and priorities in low-income countries.* Oxford, Oxford University Press.

De Vries, J. & Van Heck, G. L. (1997) The World Health Organization Quality of Life Assessment Instrument (WHOQOL-100): Validation study with the Dutch version. *European Journal of Psychological Assessment.* 13(3), pp.164–178.

Diener, E., Ng, W., Harter, J. & Arora, R. (2010) Wealth and happiness across the world: Material prosperity predicts life evaluation, whereas psychosocial prosperity predicts positive feelings. *Journal of Personality and Social Psychology.* 99(1), pp.52–61.

Diener, E., Emmons, R. A., Larsen, R. J., & Griffin, S. (1985) The Satisfaction With Life scale. *Journal of Personality Assessment.* 49, pp.71–75.

DOH (2014) *Wellbeing and why it matters to health*. London, Department of Health. Available from: https://www.gov.uk/government/publications/wellbeing-and-health-policy [Accessed 10 March 2017].

Foresight (2008) *Foresight Mental Capital and Wellbeing Project, mental capital and wellbeing: Making the most of ourselves in the 21st century*. Final Project Report. London, Government Office for Science. Available from: https://www.gov.uk/government/uploads/system/uploads/attachment_data/file/292450/mental-capital-wellbeing-report.pdf [Accessed 10 May 2017].

Grenville-Cleave, B. (2012) *Positive psychology: A practical guide*. London, Icon Books.

Hacking, I. (1995) *Rewriting the soul: Multiple personality and the science of memory*. Princeton, NJ, Princeton University Press.

Hallam, R. S. (2009) *Virtual selves, real persons: A dialogue across disciplines*. Cambridge, Cambridge University Press.

Harré, R. (1998) *The singular self*. London, Sage.

Hatch, S. L., Harvey, S. B. & Maughan, B. (2010) A developmental-contextual approach to understanding mental health and wellbeing in early adulthood. *Social Science and Medicine*. 70(2), pp.261-68.

Hollon, S. D. & DeRubeis, R. J. (2009) Mediating the effects of cognitive therapy for depression, *Cognitive Behavior Therapy*. 38, pp.43–47.

Jahoda, M. (1958) *Current concepts of positive mental health*. New York, Basic Books.

Johnson, J., Wood, A. M., Gooding, P., Taylor, P. J. & Tarrier, N. (2011) Resilience to suicidality: The buffering hypothesis. *Clinical Psychology Review*. 31(4), pp.563–591.

Keyes, C. L. M. (2007) Promoting and protecting mental health as flourishing. *American Psychologist*. 62(2), pp.95–108.

Kinderman, P., Schwannauer, M., Pontin, E. & Tai, S. (2011) The development and validation of a general measure of well-being: The BBC well-being scale. *Qualitative Life Research*. 20, pp.1035–1042.

Layard, R. & Clark, D. M. (2014) *Thrive: The power of evidence-based psychological therapies*. London, Allen Lane.

Muraven, M., & Baumeister, R. F. (2000) Self-regulation and depletion of limited resources: Does self-control resemble a muscle? *Psychological Bulletin*, 126(2), pp.247–259.

NHS (2006) Wellbeing self assessment. Available from: https://www.nhs.uk/tools/documents/self_assessments_js/assessment.html?XMLpath=/tools/documents/self_assessments_js/packages/&ASid=43&syndicate= [Accessed 14 November 2017].

ONS (2013) *Measuring national wellbeing: What matters most to personal well-being?* London, Office for National Statistics. Available from: http://webarchive.nationalarchives.gov.uk/20160105160709/http://www.ons.gov.uk/ons/dcp171766_312125.pdf [Accessed 10 November 2016].

Orford, J. (2008) *Community psychology: Challenges, controversies and emerging consensus*. Chichester, Wiley.

Pavot, W. & Diener, E. (2009) Review of the satisfaction with life scale. In: Diener, E. (ed.) *Assessing well-being: The collected works of Ed Diener*. New York, Springer, pp.101–117.

PHE (2015) *Attitudes to mental health problems and mental wellbeing: Findings from the 2015 British Social Attitudes survey*. Public Health England. Available from: www.bsa.natcen.ac.uk/latest-report/british-social-attitudes-33/mental-health.aspx [Accessed 10 May 2017].

Platt, J., Prins, S., Bates, L. & Keyes, K. (2016) Unequal depression for equal work? How the wage gap explains gendered disparities in mood disorders. *Social Science and Medicine*. 149, pp.1–8.

Ryan, R. M. & Deci, E. L. (2001) On happiness and human potentials: A review of research on hedonic and eudaimonic well-being. *Annual Review of Psychology*. 52, pp.141–66.

Ryff, C. D. & Singer, B. H. (2008) Know thyself and become what you are: A eudaimonic approach to psychological well-being. *Journal of Happiness Studies*. 9, pp.13–39.

Salter, A. (1949) *Conditioned reflex therapy: The direct approach to the reconstruction of personality*. New York, Creative Age Press.

Schrank, B., Woppmann, A., Sibitz, M. I., & Lauber, C. (2011) Development and validation of an integrative scale to assess hope. *Health Expectations*. 14(4), pp.417–428.

Schwarz, N. (1999) Self-reports: How the questions shape the answers. *American Psychologist*. 54(2), pp.93–105.

Schwartz, A., Goldiamond, I. & Howe, M. W. (1975) *Social casework: A behavioral approach*. New York, Columbia University Press.

Seligman, M. (2011) *Flourish: A new understanding of happiness and well-being – and how to achieve them*. London, Nicholas Brealey.

Seligman, M. E. P. (2002) *Authentic happiness: Using the new positive psychology to realize your potential for lasting fulfillment*. New York, Free Press.

Sen, A. (1999) *Development as freedom*. Oxford, Oxford University Press.

Stafford, M. et al. (2015) Childhood environment and mental wellbeing at age 60–64 Years: Prospective evidence from the MRC National Survey of Health and Development. *PLoS ONE*. 10(6), e0126683.

Tennant, R. et al. (2007) The Warwick-Edinburgh Mental Well-being Scale (WEMWBS): Development and UK validation, *Health and Quality of Life Outcome*. 5, p.63.

Watkins, E. R. (2009) Depressive rumination: Investigating mechanisms to improve cognitive behavioural treatments, *Cognitive Behaviour Therapy*. 38, pp.8–14.

Weich, S. et al. (2011) Mental well-being and mental illness: Findings from the Adult Psychiatric Morbidity Survey for England 2007, *British Journal of Psychiatry*. 199(1), pp.23–28.

Westerhof, G. J. & Keyes, C. L. M. (2010) Mental illness and mental health: The two continua model across the lifespan. *Journal of Adult Development*. 17(2), pp.110–119.

White, R. G., Imperiale, M. G. & Perera, E. (2016) The Capabilities Approach: Fostering contexts for enhancing mental health and wellbeing across the globe. *Globalization and Health*. 12, p.16.

WHO (n.d.) *Constitution of WHO: Principles*. Available from: www.who.int/about/mission/en/ [Accessed 10 May 2017].

WHO (2004) *Promoting mental health: Concepts, emerging evidence, practice*. Available from: www.who.int/mental_health/evidence/en/promoting_mhh.pdf [Accessed 10 May 2017].

Wood, A. M. & Tarrier, N. (2010) Positive clinical psychology: A new vision and strategy for integrated research and practice, *Clinical Psychology Review*. 30(7), pp.819–829.

8

A FUTURE WITHOUT THE CONCEPT OF MENTAL ILLNESS

I have invited the reader to imagine a future in which we could confront our woes without a concept of mental illness. The concept explains very little and has obscured the search for causes and solutions. The task of confronting a woe is both personal and shared. The default expectation seems to be that adults who have no obvious impediments should accept primary responsibility for dealing with whatever befalls them. Woes do, of course, elicit help and support from friends and family, and sometimes from whole communities and the State. So-called mental illness has been taken to be one of those impediments that can account for a person's failure to overcome their woes or to adjust their behaviour when they cause woes for others. Once a person is judged to be mentally ill, it paves the way for access to specialist help and to an intervention funded by the State. Under the umbrella of health and welfare, the State perceives that it has an obligation to relieve woes and foster well-being.

Abolishing the concept of mental illness would not remove the role of the State, but it would weaken one of the ideological pillars of a 'mental health service'. With regard to physical health, the State steps in to mitigate risks and treat illness. People are expected to adopt a healthy lifestyle but are rarely blamed for becoming physically ill, even when blame would not be out of place. With regard to mental health, the obligations of the individual and the State are rarely stated with any clarity. Public attitudes to policies governing mental health and welfare depend to some extent on how much a person is expected to rely on their own resources. There is criticism, for instance, of a 'nanny State' that steps in to assist the woeful. One effect of assimilating woes into a concept of health, and attributing them to biomedical disorders, is to shape the nature of the State's perceived obligations. As illnesses or diseases, woes are likely to be seen as misfortunes rather than as foreseeable and preventable. In reality, there are many causes of common woes that could be mitigated without surrendering the idea that ultimate responsibility for living well lies with the individual (Thoits, 2010).

It is becoming increasingly clear that physical illness and so-called mental illness share many causes in common (PHE, 2017). From the perspective of prevention, the division between them is difficult to maintain. Where it is possible to address and prevent the psychosocial causes of woes directly, this is clearly preferable to mopping up their negative consequences. In the case of physical health, it is not controversial to adopt a sensible diet, to exercise, or to desist from smoking. Similarly, many woes described as mental ill-health are potentially preventable. Some of them do have a primary somatic cause, and in this case they are candidates for a biomedical intervention. However, when somatic dysfunction/impairment is secondary to psychosocial causes, I have suggested that it is preferable to tackle the latter rather than take a biomedical approach.

The medicalisation of woes has shaped public policy in many ways. The invented status of 'mental illness' is rarely questioned; these so-called illnesses are collections of 'symptoms' that have not yet been validated as mental or bodily disorders by the discovery of detectable processes that could explain their origin. Criteria for psychiatric diagnoses are determined by committees who convene at intervals to produce manuals that organise various kinds of observation and theoretical opinion into a system to which the contributing experts can (mostly) agree. Psychiatric manuals can be compared to the 'standard operating procedures' that any technical, bureaucratic, or military organisation finds it necessary to devise. In this respect, they have been highly successful in achieving their purpose, and their influence is global. New disorders are invented and others are deleted over the course of time. Bulimia (binge eating and purging) became an official disorder in the American *Diagnostic and Statistical Manual* (*DSM*) in 1980; in 1987, homosexuality was removed from the *DSM*. The list of disorders has been growing steadily over the past fifty years. Their 'existence' allows them to be counted, so that figures for incidence and prevalence can be published and compared across countries and tabulated against various social parameters.

In practice, the concept of mental illness decontextualises woes so that their psychosocial origins and maintenance are obscured. Medicalisation also amounts to a professional territorial claim that has the effect of shunting competing perspectives into a secondary or subordinate position. Through mystification, people are induced to surrender control to experts, leaving them effectively in the position of bystanders who have little to contribute. The terminology of 'illness', 'disorder', and 'psychopathology' signifies a departure from what is thought to lie within the competence of family, peers, lay advisers, or the larger community.

Psychiatric diagnostic criteria have been sufficiently plausible to convince scientific researchers to investigate the precursors and psychosocial effects of woes defined in this manner. As a result, research has been channelled in unhelpful ways. Some researchers have developed 'disorder-specific' causal models but the latter usually end up by redefining the disorder. Other researchers, seeing less use for psychiatric diagnosis, have developed 'trans-diagnostic models'. These research strategies accommodate to medicalisation without eradicating its influence.

Medicalisation has proved useful in creating a structure for the organised delivery of services funded under the umbrella of health. Degrees of disorder, measured in terms of number or severity of 'symptoms', now constitute the basic unit of input and output for a health production process. Without this manner of parcelling up woes, 'treatment' would have to be replaced by something much more diffuse and difficult to pin down for managerial purposes.

One positive effect of abolishing the concept of mental illness would be to direct attention towards a society-wide conception of causation. This, in turn, should generate policies designed to prevent adversities known to be harmful to well-being. In fact, some attempts to reduce stress and raise well-being have already been piloted and shown to be cost-effective in economic analyses (Lomas, 2015). Another consequence of abolition would be to render as fairly meaningless the call for parity of funding between 'physical' and 'mental' health. With respect to prevention, the two areas are becoming less distinguishable, and therefore parity does not need special pleading. With respect to 'treatment', I have argued that the concept of mental illness is a flawed basis for organising interventions.

The life circumstances that potentially cause woes are diverse and difficult to classify. Adversity affects everybody, as well as tipping some people over the edge into long-term distress or problems that are resistant to change. Parity of funding for mental health is usually interpreted as a call for increased resources to treat disorders. The fact that calls for parity have gone unanswered for so long is probably due to a tacit recognition that a policy founded on the treatment of disorders would require a bottomless pit of resources. In place of a vague notion of mental health, it would seem preferable to fractionate the field into different woes and deal with them according to what is known about their causes and potential solutions. When analysed contextually, it should become clearer how responsibility should be distributed between the individual, community, and State. In so far as woes arise as a result of misfortune, a person's bad choices, their conflicts and moral dilemmas, these are not the kind of cause that the State is in much position to prevent or influence directly. However, the moral, existential, and political dimensions of woes would be exposed with greater clarity in the absence of the mystification generated by viewing woes as illnesses. Resistance to medicalisation has stemmed, in part, from the imposition of inappropriate analyses of woeful situations.

Medicalisation, social policy, and alternatives

Before commenting on views expressed in some recent UK mental health policy documents, I will describe a few innovative developments that respond to woes in new ways. While some have a grass-roots origin, others have been developed by mental health professionals working against the grain. In Chamberlin's terminology (see Chapter 6), the latter are supportive or partnership arrangements.

When envisioning alternatives to a State-provided mental health system, it is necessary to recognise the complex relationship between grass-roots and professional knowledge. On the one hand, a woeful person ought to be in the best position to know what their woe is and to generate solutions for resolving it. On the other hand, professional knowledge and expertise disseminated over the past century has had a profound effect on people's understanding of how they end up in a state of distress or feel unable to resolve their problems. Social scientists, the media, and self-help books have exerted a huge influence on public awareness. This has often had an enlightening effect, encouraging people to solve their own problems or seek advice as appropriate. The professions have also undoubtedly contributed to our knowledge of how to bring about change in unwanted habits and distressing emotions. This knowledge is publicly available, and people do not necessarily have to consult anyone to make use of it.

However, professional knowledge has also shaped public discourse about woes in ways that perpetuate mystification. For instance, charitable and voluntary sector organisations in the field of mental health often adhere to medical terminology. In this way, they can prove to be an obstacle to change. As so many activists in the survivor/ex-service-user movement have argued, it is important that those in need should have the power to define what those needs are, and to exert an influence over the resources for meeting them.

The need for a fundamental rethink of the requirements of a 'mental health service' has come from both service-users and professionals. Beresford and colleagues sum up the views expressed by a large sample of service-users who took part in focus groups: 'Some service users felt that a more social approach to mental health issues was unlikely to make major progress so long as the welfare (*disability*) benefits system continued to be based effectively on a medical model' (Beresford et al., 2016: 53). Participants in the survey were not so much opposed to medication as medicalisation. Many criticised anti-stigma campaigns because of their acceptance of an illness model. Participants welcomed opportunities to talk and think about mental health in a different way, recognising that there was no one way forward: 'People are different and there needs to be a range of different approaches so that people can find something that works for them' (ibid.: 43). These opinions are similar to those expressed by service-users 25 years ago (Rogers and Pilgrim, 1993).

Professionals have aired radical opinion in books such as *Prevention through political action and social change* (Joffe and Albee, 1981). Two psychiatrists, Mosher and Burti (1994), have written convincingly about alternatives to present services. There are now numerous examples of innovative community-based alternatives to statutory services (see Maisel, 2016; Beckwith, Bliuc, and Best, 2016). Many of the organisations that lobby on behalf of a particular woe (and in some cases offer services) construct their advice and devise self-help material on the basis of published research, and in conjunction with professionals.

Despite these positive professional influences, it ought to be axiomatic that a person in a woeful position should be the prime mover when deciding how to comprehend and respond to it. This seems to be Szasz's position based on his libertarian philosophy. Joffe and Albee (1981) take issue with Szasz's contention that 'he prefers to let people make their own decisions about matters that do not injure others rather than coerce them by means of religious, penal, or psychiatric sanctions' (1981: 3). Joffe and Albee suggest that Szasz should argue with as much passion about the coercion of the weak and powerless as he does about psychiatric coercion. However, political weakness and powerlessness are often a consequence of naming, leading to a concomitant loss of human rights. An example of beneficial re-labelling (in this case, coming largely from advocates and carers) is how the lives of 'imbeciles' and 'retardates' were changed over the course of the last century by policies inspired by the concept of social role valorisation (Osburn, 2006). As Szasz (1981) puts it this way:

> The idea of 'preventing psychopathology' thus comes down to this. First, we must examine the contents of various moral codes and the specific behavioral repertoires they promote or inhibit. Second, we must decide whether or not using coercion to enforce such codes is desirable, and if so under what circumstances and in what ways.
>
> *Szasz, 1981: 33*

Szasz's reference to 'various moral codes' follows from his belief that problems in living are created by the decisions a person makes (or fails to make). Although I have not fully endorsed this view, Szasz draws attention to the fact that medical labelling is not a neutral act but reflects practices that take a moral position.

Abolition of the concept of mental illness is unlikely to lead to complacency about the causes of woes. The fading away of talk about witches and devils did not lead to a loss of interest in social reform. Abolition only implies removing an attribution of mental illness as grounds for interpreting, labelling, or coercing the woeful. That many people are content to describe themselves as mentally ill is beside the point. Persons in the past have believed themselves to be witches (and a few still do), but this is not a reason to cling on to a belief in witchcraft.

Mental health professionals in a service economy

A very large number of people are employed in mental health services, welfare agencies, and associated industries. They all cater to the needs of the woeful in one way or another. Amongst them are health professionals who Susskind and Susskind include within a larger group of 'human experts'. These authors define a professional as someone who possesses useful knowledge and skills that lay people do not. Professionals generate new ideas and methods, and 'curate the knowledge over which they have mastery' (2015: 16). Entry into a profession is limited to those with appropriate credentials, and entrants are then licensed and regulated for ethical standards and competency. To a large extent, a profession sets its own values and standards.

In the mental health sector, the independent professional has largely given way to managed services whose *raison d'être* departs from the tradition of consulting an expert. The professional has become an employee with job security, and she or he has less control over the nature of the service they provide. The independent practitioner who is paid by third parties also surrenders a portion of their freedom to act in light of their own skills and values. Mosher and Burti point out the significance of the terms used to identify the recipient:

> The first step in the analysis of a request is to question who the real customer is. The term *customer* is currently used to define the real purchaser of the intervention requested. In private practice the patient is generally also the customer: He goes to a professional and asks for help by himself. The patient is a client. In public mental health this rarely happens. Instead, in many cases the patient is brought to the attention of the agency *by others*, often unwillingly: the patient and the customer are not the same person.
>
> *Mosher and Burti, 1994: 20; original emphasis*

The structure of present services is shaped by psychiatric definitions of woes and official guidance on an 'evidence-base' for treatment. Medical terminology has been adopted as the accepted *modus operandi*. The self-correcting influence of the professions has begun to wither as general managers take over the running of services. Managers maintain that they follow best practice, but the latter reflects a selective interpretation of the evidence. Managers also have to translate policies devised by their funders (the State or health insurers) into a workable arrangement of resources on the ground, with a constant eye on costs and demonstrable outcomes. Consequently, there is a filtering of professional expertise, which can lead to a narrowing of perspective and exaggerated claims for the methods adopted. Medicalisation is entrenched in State services and private enterprise, and so any move towards a deeper appreciation of the psychosocial causes of so-called mental illness would inevitably encounter strong resistance.

McKnight has railed against the appropriation of care by a service economy, stating: 'Revolutions begin when people who are defined as problems achieve the power to redefine the problem' (1995: 16). He argues from the position that the power to label people as deficient and view them as in need is a basic tool of oppression in modern industrialised societies. According to him, the natural problem-solving capacities of citizens are usurped by professionals whose ministrations are disabling.

While it is true that professionals have, in the main, become employees of the service sector, it is also the case that professionals have worked collaboratively and in support of grass-roots organisations. McKnight's attack on professionals does not discriminate between the different roles they could perform. Susskind and Susskind (2015) offer a rather different criticism of the professions. They argue that traditional practices are old-fashioned, inefficient, and unnecessarily exclusive and expensive. McKnight (1995: 21) believes that the professions cannot be reformed whereas Susskind and Susskind are of the opinion that professional practice could be modernised in order to serve the public better. They suggest that there is nothing unique about specialist knowledge, that methods are often antiquated and inscrutable, that professionals should not be left to regulate themselves, and that much of their work need not take on a bespoke character. Their main recommendations can be summed up as follows: routinise those parts of the work that can be performed better by using dedicated software, communicate via the Internet and take advantage of its data resources, employ paraprofessionals in much of the face-to-face work or for carrying out simpler tasks, decompose tasks into their components, and multi-source where this is advantageous. Susskind and Susskind anticipate a time when:

> It is entirely conceivable that systems will eventually be better than people in gauging the mood of human beings. More, by using advanced speech synthesis (ensuring a kindly voice perhaps), drawing on a large database of triggers and appropriate responses (a collection of *mots justes*), and by reference to users' psychological and emotional profiles, it is foreseeable that machines will be equipped to respond to their users in a manner that would *appear* to be *more* empathetic than a human being.
>
> *Susskind and Susskind, 2015: 252; original emphasis*

These developments in the mental health sector are very close to having been realised. Para-professionals began to be employed at least fifty years ago (e.g. Marks et al., 1976) and 'digital' therapy (e-therapy) is now commonplace and delivered with minimal human involvement (Hallam, 2015a; Pugh et al., 2014). In a typical managed care system, woes are broken down into individual components, each requiring its own learning module or specialist. Services are provided according to strict geographical location, age group, or problem type. The nature of a problem and the effectiveness of help are defined in terms dictated by the service provider.

Susskind and Susskind (2015) may be right to believe that a great deal of face-to-face professional expertise could be delivered better by dedicated software when it is fed the right sort of data. However, a distinction can be been drawn between personal services and other types of profession. The former aim to bring about 'changes in the personality or body of the client' (Halmos, 1970: 22), and this focuses attention on the quality of the client–professional relationship. Susskind and Susskind's vision appears to assume that all professional skills are essentially technical. But human problems entail moral dilemmas for which there is no one correct solution. When a person's problem amounts to not knowing what the problem is, it would be difficult to design software that would ask relevant questions. In these scenarios, technical means/ends solutions have little place. Moreover, problems often involve other people – employers, neighbours, and communities – for whom there is no 'right' solution that will please everyone. At present, an open-ended conversation with a person or between a group of persons is probably the best means we have to resolve problems of this type.

Susskind and Susskind's (2015) recommendations for professional practice depend on the employment of technical terms, of which a medical vocabulary is one example. A belief in the existence of psychiatric disorders leads to an assumption that they can be counted and eliminated. This takes the definition of woes out of the hands of the woeful. On the basis that people do want their woes attended to, Halmos (1970: 25) predicted, nearly fifty years ago, that there would be a large expansion of the personal professions, and he was correct. However, he was wrong to suppose that a personal ethos would spread to the non-personal category of profession; a trend in the opposite direction seems to have occurred.

Many employees of mental health or welfare services are not professionals as defined by Susskind and Susskind. Expertise is transmitted as packages of care that are delivered according to a set protocol. Even if an employee is capable of implementing a more creative and tailored service, budget constraints, fixed eligibility criteria, or prescribed allocations of service time will probably prevent it. Moreover, in the UK, the ethical standards and competence of many mental health workers are no longer regulated by the professions to which they belong but by quasi-governmental bodies run by lay administrators. It seems inevitable that this approach to regulation will stifle a profession's ability to curate its own knowledge, to reflect on the ethical implications of practice, and to innovate new solutions.

To summarise, psychiatric diagnosis has fulfilled a need to pin down and classify distress so that it can be acted upon within a managed rule-based system. This has meant that complex woeful situations have not been given the subtle analysis they deserve, bearing in mind that a tailored, negotiated, and pragmatic response is often required when weighing up what to do. It has been argued that diagnosis should be replaced by a process of individual problem formulation (BPS, 2011; Hallam, 2013). Although it is true that medical diagnosis involves formulation and contains elements of negotiation and patient choice, the latter need to be far more prominent in the resolution of so-called mental health problems. Present methods of management in the mental health system would have to change radically to accommodate a substantial degree of individual formulation.

In practice, the process of formulation may be more or less complex. The moral and existential dimensions of a person's woe may be large or small, and may be appreciated by the woeful to a greater or lesser extent or not at all. People often resort to quick fixes because they are unwilling to take a broader view or because the barriers to change seem insurmountable. The expectation of those who are willing to address problems in depth (with peers or with a professional adviser) is that a new understanding of their woe will to some extent dissolve their distress. Resistance to medicalisation has nearly always been accompanied by a call to raise consciousness about a wide range of issues from the most general (e.g. philosophical, spiritual, political) to the most mundane (e.g. how to fill in a form to apply for a benefit). Ultimately, it is the individual who experiences their woe most acutely, and it is rare that a one-size-fits-all solution is ever available.

Shared conversations

Where possible, it seems desirable that a shared conversation and negotiation should take the place of a rigid package of care for a pre-defined problem. The prototypical professional consultation is a person talking confidentially to an expert who diagnoses a suspected problem and offers to help to solve it. This was the model for verbal psychotherapy when it first developed within medicine, and it continues to be the way most 'common mental disorders' are dealt with. Individual therapy may at times extend to family members, but family therapy is usually regarded as a separate specialisation. Therapy in groups is difficult to organise within a State-funded service unless its members reside in the same place. Groups are easier to provide outside normal working hours by independent practitioners or voluntary organizations. The need that grass-roots movements have managed to fill is the opportunity for groups of people, sharing similar problems, to get together to discuss their concerns.

In its most extreme form, medicalisation removes from the so-called patient the human right to be spoken to as a person. Buck-Zerchin writes about her 'treatment' in Germany as follows:

> I experienced five different psychiatric hospitals from 1936 to 1959 with 23 professors of psychiatry, medical directors, senior physicians and their assistants. They all subscribed to a genetically caused, meaningless and incurable schizophrenia. As a result, I didn't experience a single conversation about the content of my psychoses or the life-crisis that led to them and certainly not about any meaningful connections.
>
> *Buck-Zerchin, 2007: 28*

Similarly, in the UK, a young man hospitalised at intervals between 1959 and 1971, only learned in 1969 that his mother's death was the result of her taking her own life (Hallam and Bender, 2011: 81). His detailed journals contain almost no reference to conversations with professionals about his life circumstances. His discovery about the cause of his mother's death was prompted by his own impulse to ask. Even then, his psychiatrist said he should ask his father about it. Only after insistent interrogation did she admit the truth. Her reluctance to disclose might have reflected her assumption that mention of upsetting realities would only make the 'fragile mad' more mad still.

These two examples are taken from a period in which medicalisation was almost completely dominant. However, the views of present-day service-users indicate that change has not yet gone far enough (Beresford, et al., 2016). Recent decades have witnessed the growth of voluntary alliances between people who feel that they have had to endure discrimination pertaining to gender, sexuality, race, disability, and madness. Shared conversations have been conducted through the written word, workshops, conferences, websites, blogs, and peer discussion. Full and frank discourse can be expected to have the following beneficial effects: acknowledgement of a person's unique story and experiences, a re-description without the use of pejorative labels, exposure to others' perspectives, critical distancing from a problem by contextualising experience, a re-examination of disowned parts of one's own experience, sharing with warm empathic others, and a decreased sense of alienation through learning that others have been through something similar. Holmes (2010) and Shaw (2013) offer examples of how local peer support groups can be established and run successfully.

Experiments in creating a different kind of conversation with so-called psychiatric patients can be traced to therapeutic communities developed during work with soldiers traumatised by their experiences during the Second World War (Main, 1946). Later on, some British anti-psychiatrists set up small communities in which traditional doctor–patient relationships were overturned. These led to other experiments with small community living arrangements supported by professionals.

In recent years, the power of conversation has been exploited in the 'open dialogue' method developed in Finland but now practised in other parts of the world (see below). In community settings, some mental health professionals have moved away from traditional models of individual therapy and have set up more accessible and informal arrangements (Holmes, 2010: 22; White, 2008).

Soteria Houses

In the 1960s, the psychiatrist R. D. Laing and his colleagues experimented with community living (situated at Kingsley Hall in London) for people diagnosed with psychosis. Madness was understood to be a meaningful (though chaotic) experience, and medication was used sparingly. This model inspired a later American experiment in the 1970s, Soteria House in San Jose, California (Mosher, Hendrix and Fort, 2004). Instead of suppressing so-called symptoms with drugs, this community house described its method as 'being with', a form of close personal contact with one or more household staff which could potentially last for hours on end. The staff developed their own non-medical terminology that suited their philosophy and values. The creation of Soteria House was, in part, a product of the counter-cultural ethos of the 1970s. However, there are current examples of Soteria Houses in the US (e.g. Vermont) and the UK (Bradford and Brighton, see Soteria Network, UK, n.d.; Pearson and Baboulene, 2016). Soteria Houses have encountered resistance, and one in Alaska was forced to close (Gottstein, 2015). The irony of this situation is that the results achieved by the Soteria approach can be justified when judged against biomedical criteria.

Carpenter and Buchanan identify methodological weaknesses in the evaluation of the Soteria project, but these are, in principle, resolvable. The bottom line is that the approach is perceived as a threat: 'Soteria House provided an early demonstration of an alternative to hospital-based care but chose ideology over influence and opposition over integration' (Carpenter and Buchanan, 2002: 579). In a more balanced review, Calton and colleagues conclude that 'the Soteria paradigm yields equal, and in certain specific areas, better results in the treatment of people diagnosed with first- or second-episode schizophrenia spectrum disorders (achieving this with considerably lower use of medication) when compared with conventional, medication-based approaches' (Calton et al., 2008: 181).

Viewed historically, it is remarkable that Soteria House was funded as a controlled experiment by the US National Institute of Mental Health (NIMH). It is now unthinkable that NIMH would fund a similar study, given the present dominance of a biomedical approach to psychosis (Abbott, 2016). It is also worth emphasising that renouncing a concept of mental illness creates a different kind of relationship between workers and residents. The intimacy of personal contact would be considered 'unprofessional' from the medical standpoint adopted by bodies that regulate the ethics and competence of mental health workers.

Open dialogue

This approach was developed in the 1980s in a generic mental health service in Lapland, where teams of workers responded to crisis situations (typically psychosis) wherever they occurred (Seikkula, 2006; Seikkula et al., 2011). The approach has since spread to many countries and is currently being evaluated in several regional NHS centres in the UK. Because it developed within a mental health service, it is important to state what makes it a non-medical intervention. First, the problem is fully contextualised (with meetings taking place in the home, work situation, or other convenient location) and the aim is to involve any person who has played a potential role in the development of a crisis or could be useful in resolving it. Meetings are held to allow participants to converse about the situation from their own perspective. Mental health professionals facilitate meetings but participation is on an equal basis. Second, the response to the crisis is immediate. Third, there is no need for a medical diagnosis or the employment of medical terminology. The meeting is an 'open dialogue', with an emphasis on listening, not on pressure to make decisions or form treatment plans. The professional members of the team may include inpatient staff. In this case, the same team operates in outpatient and inpatient settings.

Although this is primarily a non-medical approach, a decision may be reached to prescribe antipsychotic medication when there is general agreement that this would be helpful. The skills of open dialogue work differ considerably from conventional methods. Staff members typically receive two years' training. The results achieved by this approach are impressive. Only about one-third of people are prescribed antipsychotic medication, and around 80 per cent return to work or are relieved of their psychotic experiences (Seikkula et al., 2011; Seikkula, Alakare and Aaltonen, 2011). The question marks hanging over the success of its transfer to traditionally run mental health services are as follows: whether an approach adopted by a generic service in a small, predominantly rural community can work as well in an urban environment; whether a highly managed and medically structured service can provide the immediacy, consistency, and continuity required; whether the unique philosophy and training for this style of work can be adopted in other settings. As Seikkula remarks: 'But what has surprised me is the enormous difficulty therapists with extensive experience in a particular therapeutic method have in adopting a dialogical way of working with clients' (2011: 185).

Hearing Voices Movement (HVM)

The HVM has been a very successful development in recent years. From its roots in the Netherlands, it has now spread across the world and is served by an international organisation, Intervoice. It began in the 1980s as a collaboration between a psychiatrist, researcher, and voice hearer (see Longden, Corstens, and Dillon, 2013). HVM works to promote acceptance and understanding of hearing voices by critiquing and reframing biomedical accounts. It seeks to replace the view that hearing voices are symptoms of serious mental illness with the idea that they can be accepted as common experiences for which there are many explanations, including prior psychological trauma (Leudar and Thomas; 2000, McCarthy-Jones, 2017). Members of HVM operate as peer support groups (there are over 180 in the UK) in which experiences can be shared in confidence, partly with the purpose of making peace with the voices or coping with them differently (Romme and Escher, 2009). Although HVM does not proscribe any person's interpretation of their voices, it is clearly unsympathetic to the view that sees them as a symptom of mental illness. HVM operates as a partnership model in Chamberlin's terms, and how its future relationship with existing services will develop remains uncertain (Corstens et al., 2014).

Community-based groupwork

Holmes (2010), an NHS clinical psychologist, set up and facilitates time-limited groups in his local community (in Shropshire, England), which are open to people who respond to local advertisements. The size of the groups is between 10–15 people. In practice, around two-thirds of the members are already involved in primary or secondary mental health services. On occasion, further group activities are inspired, planned, and coordinated by group members without professional involvement. Holmes describes the group ethos as 'collaborative conversation', meaning that members are collaborators and peers who are willing to suspend pre-judging others and are open to different points of view. Initially at least, the groups are facilitated by a skilled group leader who is able to ensure that discussion remains dialogical and more or less on theme. The work, although funded by the NHS, is non-medical in the sense that members do not have to register as service-users or be entered onto a database. There is no entry criterion or assessment process. The topics for group discussion are not psychiatric disorders or 'coping skills'. Instead, dialogue is directed towards the contextualisation of people's problems, learning from others, and mutual support. There is also a focus on the effects of oppression and disempowerment. Groups have dealt with issues such as 'understanding depression' and 'thinking about medication'. Groups of a more informal nature have involved 'walking and talking' and 'therapeutic journal writing'.

Community-based approaches of this kind do not fit easily into the managed delivery of services that requires adherence to evidence-based protocols, registration of service-users, recording of 'episodes of care', obligatory risk assessments, and payment by results. As Holmes observes (2010: 273), managers of health and social care services are reluctant to surrender control to local people with the power to decide how they might be helped.

Community-wide initiatives

A similar but more wide-ranging and multi-levelled service, also led by an NHS clinical psychologist, was developed in Glasgow, Scotland (White, 2008). The striking features of this service were the use of advertising to reach as many people as possible, removing obstacles to accessibility, the diversity of different media employed in delivery, e.g. group meetings, classes, workshops, self-help material downloadable from a website or available in libraries, 30-minute time slots for advice (face-to-face or by phone), collaboration with physical health services, and staff training offered to various organisations. If a person required a more intensive intervention, they were 'stepped-up' to the level required. Materials were made available in translation for different language groups and contacts were made with leaders of ethnic groups within the city. White left the service in 2013 and since then it has reverted back to a more conventional role of providing therapy in response to GP referrals (White, 2017, personal communication). In other words, the aims of direct community involvement and greater access have been dropped. Although individual therapy satisfies an important need for people with intransigent problems, it is not credible to suppose that this model can be provided economically at a population-wide level.

Continuing with the same mental health policies

I conclude by commenting on a number of UK policy recommendations published in recent years. My intention is to confront rhetoric with reality and to reconcile, where possible, the arguments presented in this book with imagined futures for 'mental health'. Problems in living can never be eliminated because life is unavoidably messy. People often fail to solve their problems or live up to their own standards; they deviate in ways that may annoy and affect others. The mess is presently swept up by society into a big heap called 'mental ill-health', a heterogeneous pile of difficulties whose only common characteristic is that those affected call out for them to be resolved, contained, and, where possible, recycled into a state of satisfactory well-being.

Official responses do not, of course, always satisfy those involved. As long as the task of sorting out mental ill-health is assigned to government officials, policy advisers, regulators, and managers, the result will be a network of arrangements resembling any other society-wide function such as transport, waste disposal, or education. A systematic approach works reasonably well for physical health because citizens have access to information upon which to make choices, and they usually trust professionals to make good decisions on their behalf. What makes the mess of mental ill-health unique is that its causes are far more opaque. The problem is compounded by myths about madness and biological causation. Furthermore, distress may be associated with a sense of failure, and a suspicion that something that could have been prevented was not, whether that something was of an intensely personal or public nature. Consequently, woes are typically charged with negative emotion (such as shame, anger, guilt, or resentment) that is preferably covered up or neutralised by a spray of disinfecting terminology. In brief, any system set up to deal with mental health as a set of discrete disorders is ill-equipped to confront the origins of problems, their variety, and the complexity of the task it faces.

The situation is not helped when policy is devised by personnel who have had relatively little first-hand experience in a face-to-face helping role. The documents discussed below often sound overly optimistic and give the impression that everything is under control. It is usually envisaged that projected changes to policy will save money, and that previously messy people will be returned to society as economically productive members.

The illusion fostered by a technical/bureaucratic approach to mental health is the prospect of producing a rational inventory of its tasks, of parcelling up people for processing by teams of workers (preferably not too highly paid), of standardising problems into distinct bundles, prescribing how they should be dealt with, and keeping tight regulatory control over costs and throughput by measuring success in terms of its own choosing.

Proctor (2015) has offered an assessment of the present mental health system by revisiting some predictions she made in 2002 about the way services were likely to develop in the UK. Actual events have confirmed her predictions with respect to trends towards standardisation, uniformity, close surveillance of 'efficiency', cost control through competitive tendering, and providers being driven by profit or 'targets' rather than humanistic values. It remains to be seen whether the present approach to 'mental health' will eventually crack under the stress of its own contradictions. This will be so if the vision of efficiency is unrealised, if staff cannot be found to service the system without unacceptable cost to themselves, and if the public shows a desire for something different.

The concept of a National Health Service free at the point of delivery is justifiably treasured by the British electorate, although what at first comes to mind in this regard is physical health. As already noted, most people are alert to potential somatic problems and they accept professional advice. If they reject it, there is the prospect of a second opinion. The consumer can at least feel in charge when defining their needs. The situation with respect to free access to a mental health service differs in important ways. A person may be reluctant to use a service bearing in mind the stigma that attaches to 'mental illness'. She or he may lack confidence that the service will in fact deal with their problem, given that there is widespread ignorance about professional roles, therapy methods, and expected outcomes. A service will almost certainly not be requested if a person senses that it entails coercion. Moreover, when the provision of a free service is predicated on the problem being one of 'illness' or 'mental disorder', this may not match the way a person perceives their woe (Thoits, 2016).

The negotiating stance of carefully listening to a person's own account of their problem is fully appreciated by most mental health professionals. If they did not listen in this way, they would soon be out of business. In this respect, the market does rule, as in other areas of life. However, as the mental health system is currently constructed, this fundamental principle is violated when it defines the needs of its consumers and restricts services to the ones it has already decided to offer. This policy is justified by appealing to a scientific evidence-base. The evidence consists chiefly of the results of randomised control trials (RCTs) that show which therapeutic method delivers the best results for a particular 'disorder' when ranked against another method or 'treatment as usual'. Over the past fifty years, this methodology has yielded valuable insights into what helps and why. However, it is limited as a guide to what to offer in practice, principally because people's problems cannot be neatly classified as disorders. Research into therapy under experimental conditions requires that unwanted sources of error be excluded. For instance, participants are excluded if they do not fit the strict criteria defining the nature of a disorder, or if they have complicating 'additional problems'. Therapy is administered according to a carefully described protocol in order that others are able to replicate it. While this type of research necessarily controls these sources of variability, it is an error to see the RCT as providing the gold standard for 'best treatment' because it does so at the expense of departing from normal field conditions. In order to show that an 'evidence-based treatment' is really effective, it is necessary to test a protocol in the field, where matching a person's problem to a specified disorder is a rather hit-or-miss process, and where staff may not be as well-trained or supervised. Even if the fit to a 'disorder' is good, there may be circumstances in a person's life that demand more immediate attention before it can be addressed (e.g. a marriage about to break down, a gambling problem, inadequate housing, or substance abuse). In practice, a therapist needs to be flexible and sufficiently skilled to adapt a protocol to a person's unique set of circumstances.

Although RCT research has also been conducted under field conditions, reproduction of 'evidence-based methods' requires that service users be appropriately 'diagnosed' using the same psychiatric criteria. The primary evaluation of outcome remains a reduction in 'pathology'.

Standardisation is fundamental to the kind of rationalisation that Susskind and Susskind (2015) recommend for the effective delivery of professional expertise. A service could not be managed easily if its employees were given the freedom to practice as they thought best. In fact, the fear of 'rogue' professionals practicing unethically or incompetently has led to legislation being passed requiring them to be registered with regulatory bodies. Complaints are handled by procedures closely resembling those used by the legal system to deal with crime. Whereas until recently most professional organisations connected to health oversaw the competence and ethical standards of their own members, this function in the UK has been surrendered to lay bodies. Given the adversarial method of investigation, any opportunity to understand why a complaint has arisen and to learn from it, is lost. In so far as regulators adopt medicalisation as the way the mental health system is supposed to operate, current practices will ossify.

One example of how medicalisation has become entrenched is a policy decision by the UK government in 2008 to invest heavily in a new workforce to 'cure' certain 'disorders'. Initially, the targets were anxiety and depression but the service (Improving Access for Psychological Therapy, IAPT) has now extended far beyond this remit. In 2015–16, IAPT services accepted 1,399,088 new referrals (IAPT, 2016). The strategy for assessing effectiveness has been to compare results with published research findings. A 'cure' has been defined as a reduction in score on a symptom questionnaire when it falls below a certain threshold. To be consistent with an appeal to an evidence base, the effectiveness of IAPT service should really have been subjected to research that randomised service-users to IAPT and to a comparison condition, but this has not been done.

IAPT can only be justified if problems and their solution can be adequately represented as the removal of symptoms, and therapeutic success actually approaches the results of 'best practice'. The evidence it has produced for its own effectiveness in 2015–16 falls short in many ways. First, approximately one-third of new referrals were not taken on for therapy, perhaps because problems did meet entry criteria or people were not interested in what was on offer. A further third of those who were accepted into therapy, attended for only one session. This group may have been offered self-help materials or decided to discontinue. The average number of sessions for those who began therapy was between three and six. The 'success rate' was as low as 38 per cent for so-called post-traumatic stress disorder and 37 per cent for so-called agoraphobia. These results are poor compared with 'gold standard' evidence. A successful outcome for 'agoraphobia' has been reported as being close to 80 per cent since the 1980s (Hofmann and Spiegel, 1999; Fava et al., 2001). The IAPT results also show that nearly two-thirds of people diagnosed with post-traumatic stress disorder do not seem to have benefited. Given the brevity of therapy, this is entirely unsurprising.

Also of some concern, the gold-standard evidence for a good outcome using cognitive behaviour therapy (CBT) to 'treat depression' seems to have become less impressive since evaluations were first undertaken in the 1980s (Johnsen and Friborg, 2015). CBT is the approach most commonly employed in IAPT. Furthermore, in a recent RCT of 'depression' under field conditions that pitted CBT against an alternative form of psychotherapy and a comparison condition (a brief psychosocial intervention), the outcome at a one-year follow-up assessment was equivalence for all conditions (Goodyer et al., 2013). It cannot be assumed that a service that purports to replicate 'best practice' is actually able to do so or that the gold standard is itself untarnished.

UK mental health policy

This final section comments on several recent UK mental health policy and consultation documents that presumably reflect the assumptions that will guide the future provision of services. The documents draw upon academic research that has clear policy implications, but the evidence is forced into a vision that does not deviate from the conviction that 'mental health' is about illnesses, that 'treatment' for the latter needs to be centrally managed more efficiently, and that tighter control is needed over costs and the monitoring of outcomes. It is assumed that strategies for responding to 'mental health' should mimic those for physical health, and that the two services should be better integrated. Relatively little consideration is given to prevention.

My principal sources for this section are (1) a consultation document published in 2009 envisaging policies for mental health projected to the year 2020 (*New Horizons, NH* – DOH, 2009), (2) a policy document, *No health without mental health* (DOH, 2011), (3) *Five Year Forward View for Mental Health* (*FYF*), produced by an independent mental health task force in 2016, whose recommendations have been accepted by the UK government (HM Government, 2017), and (4) a task force review of children's mental health called *Future in mind: Promoting, protecting and improving our children and young people's mental health and wellbeing* (*FIM* – DOH, 2015).

The WHO *Comprehensive Mental Health Action Plan 2013* (WHO, 2013; Saxena and Setoya, 2014) resembles UK policy with respect to its emphasis on effective governance, an evidence base, and the routine collection and reporting of 'a core set of mental health indicators'. However, the WHO shows greater concern for human rights and the empowerment of persons. These concerns are directed towards the 'mentally disordered', who are seen as a disabled social out-group. One of the WHO recommendations is expressed as follows: 'protection, promotion and respect for the rights of persons with mental disorders including the need to avoid stigmatization of persons with mental disorders' (WHO, 2013, point 2b).

I have grouped my comments under several headings: (1) perpetuation of the myth of mental illness, (2) optimism about progress, (3) structural requirements of managed systems, (4) neglect of a wider perspective on well-being, (5) government regulation of the mental health workforce, and (6) a lack of direction in child policy.

Perpetuation of the illness myth

New Horizons (*NH*) asserts that by 2020 'people will know that mental health problems can affect anyone, at any time, and they will also understand that these problems have causes and can be treated, just like physical illnesses' (2009: 5). The sense conveyed here is that 'mental illness' descends out of the blue, as if one has contracted a virus and no one could have seen it coming. It's just a touch of something that the doctor will fix. This degree of optimism is incomprehensible in light of research evidence cited later in the same document to the effect that 'between a quarter and a half of mental health problems in adults are potentially preventable through treatment during childhood and adolescence' (ibid.: 30).

The word 'treatment' in this quotation is one way in which the myth of mental illness is perpetuated. The document states that: 'An estimated 60 to 70 per cent of children and young people who experience mental health problems have not had appropriate interventions at a sufficiently early age' (ibid.: 37). It is not clear whether the changed language (intervention rather than treatment) is meant to imply that 'treatment' is not always appropriate. If it were to be true that appropriate interventions could (by good fortune) be provided, and that conditions affecting children adversely could be picked up and addressed, then the reader might reasonably assume that attending to present deficiencies would lead to a hopeful outlook for 'adult mental health'. In reality, despite the attempts of welfare services to detect and curb maltreatment, much of it is probably missed. If detected, there is little sign at present that any response to it would be adequate (see below).

Optimism that progress is being made

NH reports a reduction in the number of people taking their own life, especially amongst young men, mental health inpatients, and prisoners. The document is right to focus on suicide because it is the leading cause of death amongst young adults in Europe (Miret et al., 2013). In the UK, the number of people taking their own life reached its lowest point around 2006, having fallen by 27 per cent since 1981. However, the number has since levelled off or increased (ONS, 2014). With regard to a reduction in suicide amongst prisoners, there is no cause for optimism. In 2016, the number of deaths by suicide in UK prisons reached its highest point since records began in 1978 (Howard League for Penal Reform, n.d.). Of some interest, there is considerable variation in death by suicide across regions of the UK. The rate was highest in London in the 1980s, but this city now returns a low rate. Whether this variation over time or place has anything to do with the services provided by the mental health system is unclear.

Diagnosed depression (of the 'major' or 'bipolar' type) is a strong risk factor for suicide with around 15–20 per cent ending their life in this way (Miret et al., 2013). For a person who is already in psychiatric care, the risk increases with severity of depressed mood, with feelings of hopelessness, and when depressed mood is combined with substance abuse and/or an additional diagnosis of personality disorder (Hawton et al., 2013). Unfortunately, few of these risk factors are very enlightening about causation. There is a hint that if we only knew what caused the 'illness' of depression, it could be prevented. Miret and colleagues (2013) lament the underfunding of brain research, as if this would provide a solution. These authors also call for greater efficiency, noting that around one-quarter to one-half of people who have attempted suicide do not attend follow-up appointments. They state that only about a third of people with a mood problem seek help from health services. It is possible that those who fail to ask for help do not do so because they are seeking a different kind of response.

It is clear that a majority of people who are liable to end their own life are invisible to the health system. Hawton and colleagues (2013) observe that in primary care, where most depression is diagnosed, approximately three-quarters of suicide deaths are of individuals who are unknown to secondary care services.

According to the WHO:

> Suicide is a complex issue and therefore suicide prevention efforts require coordination and collaboration among multiple sectors of society, including the health sector and other sectors such as education, labour, agriculture,

> business, justice, law, defense, politics, and the media. These efforts must be comprehensive and integrated as no single approach alone can make an impact on an issue as complex as suicide.
>
> *WHO, 2017*

The clear implication seems to be that a 'single approach', such as regarding suicide as an issue of 'mental health', does not provide grounds for optimism.

Managerialism and mental health indicators

Management systems modelled on business practice are bound to look for what they consider to be plausible indicators of better or worse mental health. In the UK, 'commissioners' contract services with 'providers'. With humility, the *NH* document notes that:

> Currently commissioners are sometimes unclear exactly what care they are buying for their population. The work to develop mental health *Payment by Results* should provide some clarity, creating a nationally consistent 'language', allowing more meaningful contracting discussions between commissioners and providers.
>
> *DOH, 2009: 104*

Although it is always possible to speak more clearly, clarity does not always equate with meaningfulness.

Five Year Forward (*FYF*) assumes that investing in new forms of delivery will be outweighed by savings across the health and care system. There will be 'a requirement to move towards accountable payment approaches in mental health which have a payment component linked to quality and outcomes'. Standard sets of measures will be developed for 'mental health conditions' in order to pave the way for 'benchmarking' (HM Government, 2017: 18).

The need for simplicity, transparency, and accountability is plain but this can only be achieved by presuming that what is messy can really be reduced to numbers, packages, and measured outputs. A centrally managed system requires this, but devolution of control to citizens and non-governmental agencies may ultimately turn out to be more effective, efficient, and flexible in the long run.

FYF recommends a working partnership with service users, their families and carers, and with local public, private, and voluntary sector organisations. Nevertheless, *FYF*'s main emphasis is on early identification of need and provision of 'evidence-based treatment', with new staff trained to work with children, psychosis, eating disorders, and the elderly. There is little sign of a let-up in cost containment or the application of a medical model: 'The majority of new services will be integrated with physical healthcare, especially primary care' (ibid.: 20). *FYF* believes that integrated services will deliver substantial savings.

With regard to the possibility of looking beyond a centrally managed system, the attitude expressed by *NH* is not very encouraging:

> Building and nurturing the resilience of individuals and communities are particularly important at this time. An example is the growth in voluntary self-help community projects that can foster people's sense of purpose and promote community cohesion. However, financial constraints also mean that service improvements will need to be self-financing, soundly evidence-based, and clearly related to local commissioning intentions, as informed by Joint Strategic Needs Assessments (JSNAs).
>
> *NH, 2009: 99*

This is an aspirational pat on the head but also a firm reminder of who is actually in control, with no practical suggestions for implementation.

Neglect of factors conducive to wellbeing

NH points to an area that is important for 'mental health', namely work and opportunities for further education and creative leisure. It states that 'work is good for mental well-being' (2009: 48). In reality, work can also be very bad for well-being and become a significant source of stress (Silcox, 2009). Attention therefore ought to be paid to the conditions in which work is undertaken (working hours, remuneration, security of employment, absence of bullying, etc.). Some employers recognise this and sign up their employees to insurance policies that cover counselling. *NH* agrees that 'Addressing employees' health and well-being makes good business sense' (ibid.: 48). It applies this advice to itself: 'The NHS aims to be a good employer by, for example, promoting healthy workplaces for professional staff' (ibid.: 49). In reality, in a period of austerity, annual increments in remuneration have not kept up with inflation. Nurses had a 14 per cent cut in pay in real terms between 2010 and 2017, and the Royal College of Nursing has been handing out hardship grants (National Health Executive, n.d.). Surveys of some groups of NHS staff show extremely worrying low levels of well-being. Healthcare professionals have amongst the highest rates of suicide for any occupational group in England and Wales. In a survey of staff well-being that included 88 per cent of workers from the NHS, around one-third reported feeling depressed in the past week either 'some of the time', 'often', or 'all of the time'. A similar proportion felt 'as if I am a failure'. Nearly 20 per cent described their job as stressful 'all of the time' (Rao et al., 2016). It is not desirable for depressed workers to be 'treating' depressed people.

With regard to other influences on well-being, *NH* expresses the opinion that:

> Adult learning influences attitudes and behaviour; it can improve skills, confidence and employment and may prevent cognitive decline . . . The National Institute of Adult Continuing Education (NIACE) aims to support and increase the number of adults participating in formal and informal learning.
>
> *NH, 2009: 50*

Since this time, many residential adult education centres have been closed and fees have risen to a level that is unaffordable except for people on a good income. Instead of creative leisure, continuing education has focused on courses to enhance students' employability. Cuts to local authority budgets have led to the closure of libraries and other community amenities.

Although *NH* makes reference to prevention at many points, such as acknowledging the role of poverty, a need to redress social inequalities, and programmes to improve employment, housing, education, and transport, the language it employs is essentially one of medical treatment. It refers to 'clinical effectiveness', 'evidence-based care pathways', 'recovery (living a life beyond illness)', and 'indicators agreed between individual clinicians and their patients'. Rather surprisingly, the reader needs to be reminded that 'It's about people who happen to use mental health services being treated as people' (ibid.: 21).

Government regulation of the mental health workforce

One *FYF* recommendation is that 'The Department of Health should consider how to introduce the regulation of psychological therapy services which are not currently inspected' (HM Government, 2017: 63). In response, the Government agreed (ibid.) but wished to consult on the idea. Its reticence probably relates to a difficulty in defining what 'therapy', a medical term, actually means in practice, and whether it can be given a legal definition. Would it, for instance, include the assessment of a person's problems, either formally or informally? If not, when would therapy officially begin and would it require a contract? Would peer discussion between service-users only count as therapy if it were led by a mental health worker? The idea of 'inspecting' human relationships sounds Orwellian, although it is in fact carried out by UK regulators of those professionals who are required by law to register if they advertise their services, or are employed by the NHS. Whether the 'inspection' of professionals is the best way to ensure protection of the public is doubtful. The investigation of complaints by means of a criminal-style examination of witnesses and written evidence is unlikely to throw much light on a breakdown of relationships between managers, service users, and mental health workers (Hallam, 2015b). In any case, apart from sexual exploitation and fraud, the rules governing working relationships are a legal grey area. To be consistent with a medical approach, a complainant who is a service user would need to have been classified as 'disordered' and to have been made worse (or harmed) by 'treatment'. This is a tall order when many forms of psychotherapy are entirely non-medical in nature, and when therapists often work in community and outreach settings where talk of 'treatment' is premature and inappropriate.

Ignoring the obvious: the maltreatment of children

The *Future in mind* document (*FIM*, DOH, 2015) illustrates how a framework of health, and the existence of a multiplicity of vested interests in a key stage of life (childhood), has led to a loss of leadership and therefore any clear idea as to who could translate new child policies into action. The *FIM* review states: 'What is needed is a fundamental shift in culture. A whole system approach is needed focusing on prevention of mental ill-health, early intervention and recovery' (ibid.: 4). A similar opinion is expressed by the Centre for Mental Health (2016): 'The implications of the evidence we have brought together are far-reaching. They point to the need for whole system ownership of and investment in children and families' mental health.'

A government minister's response to *FIM* was to announce that a new national survey of children's mental health had been commissioned (with what purpose is unclear) and that, amongst other initiatives, there had been investment in a digital app for children to record their own mental health histories. The minister referred to efforts being made to change attitudes 'so that for the next generation, the taboo of mental ill-health is removed' (DOH, 2016). There is little sign, therefore, of de-medicalisation or a serious commitment to prevention.

This is surprising given the recognition in sections of the documents (cited earlier) that responding to maltreatment in childhood is a key to success in efforts to prevent later problems. *NH* states that: 'Some 20 per cent of children in the U.K. experience some form of physical, emotional or sexual abuse' (2009: 35). There is strong evidence that an abusive childhood bodes very badly for future well-being (Greenfield and Marks, 2010; McElroy and Hevey, 2014; Mersky, Topitzes and Reynolds, 2013; Pollak, 2016; Read et al., 2014; Stafford et al., 2015; Maniglio, 2010, 2012; Cecil et al., 2017). *FIM* estimates that nearly 10 per cent of children between the ages of 5 and 16 are suffering from a 'mental disorder'. The implication of these findings is that it would be wise to invest heavily in prevention and early intervention.

There are certainly difficulties in translating policy into action because the interested parties include the children themselves, their parents and carers, nurseries, schools, health visitors, general practitioners, primary and secondary medical and mental healthcare specialists, local social workers, and youth workers. The chief organisational problem seems to be one of communication and integration:

> They [i.e. all involved] want to do the right thing, but have not necessarily been equipped to play their part or been provided with clear access routes to expertise and for referring to targeted and specialist support. Professionals working in child and adolescent mental health services are equally aware of the challenges that come from balancing identified need with available resource.
>
> *DOH, 2015: 32*

A child's problem might be first detected by neighbours, teachers, or the police, rather than parents or carers, especially where the concern is neglect, violence, physical or sexual abuse, or bullying. If the call for help begins with a child, young person, or their parents/carers, *FIM* states that:

> . . . they need clearer awareness of how to recognise when they might have a mental health problem as well as where and how to get help, clarity about

> what help is available, what might happen when they access it, and what to do while they are waiting.
>
> *Ibid.*: 39

Unfortunately, it is unclear whose role it is to commission and oversee the necessary resources. Local authorities have statutory responsibilities but they do not have ring-fenced budgets and do not necessarily see children's emotional well-being as their core business. Local NHS clinical commissioning groups (CCGs) are juggling physical health priorities at the same time. Schools may not have the expertise, time, or support they need. The Early Intervention Foundation estimates the cost to the UK economy of late interventions into childhood difficulties as being £17 billion annually (EIF, 2016).

The situation appears to have worsened since the earlier *NH* document had mentioned the existence of 'over 3,000 Sure Start Children's Centres', promoting 'integrated health and related services, delivered by well-trained professionals, whose work in their local communities will include mental health and well-being' (*NH*, 2009: 34).

Despite plans to increase the number of Sure Start centres at that time, it has been reported that 350 have closed since 2010 (Walker, 2017). It is alleged by a former health minister that money earmarked for children and young people has been diverted to plug holes in budgets for other priorities (Sharman, 2017).

Summary

Medicalisation has shaped the structure and functions of mental health services, leading to a neglect of the social causes of woes and non-medical approaches. However, the relationship between expert knowledge and grass-roots opinion (and perception of need) is a complex one. Furthermore, the traditional nature of the professions has changed, and present mental health services are led by managers whose priorities are at variance with the aims and values of a personal helping relationship. It is argued that a managed technical approach to 'mental health' fails to appreciate that woes often need to be understood as the product of a unique set of circumstances that are contextually determined. Some examples of innovative alternatives to current practice are outlined. These have generally involved professionals working in partnership with woeful individuals or with grass-roots organisations. A review of several recent UK mental health policy documents concludes that the assumptions upon which they are based cannot serve as the foundation of an approach that is likely to prove effective or sustainable.

References

Abbott, A. (2016) U.S. mental health chief: Psychiatry must get serious about mathematics. *Scientific American*. 28 October.

Beckwith, M., Bliuc, A. & Best, D. (2016) What the recovery movement tells us about prefigurative politics. *Journal of Social and Political Psychology*. 4(1). Available from: https://jspp.psychopen.eu/index.php/jspp/article/view/548/html [Accessed 10 August 2017].

Beresford, P., Perring, R., Nettle, M. & Wallcraft, J. (2016) *From mental illness to a social model of madness and distress.* Published by Shaping Our Lives. Available from: www.shapingourlives.org.uk/wp-content/uploads/2016/05/FROM-MENTAL-ILLNESS-PDF-2.pdf [Accessed 10 May 2017].

BPS (2011) *Good practice guidelines on the use of psychological formulation.* Leicester, British Psychological Society, Division of Clinical Psychology. Available from: www.bps.org.uk/system/files/Public%20files/DCP/cat-842.pdf [Accessed 10 May 2017].

Buck-Zurchin, D. S. (2007) Seventy years of coercion in psychiatric institutions, experienced and witnessed. In: Stastny, P. & Lehmann, P. (eds.) *Alternatives beyond psychiatry.* Berlin, Peter Lehmann Publishing, pp. 19–28.

Calton, T., Ferriter, M., Huband, N. & Spandler, H. (2008) A systematic review of the Soteria paradigm for the treatment of people diagnosed with schizophrenia. *Schizophrenia Bulletin*, 34(1), pp.181–192.

Carpenter, W. T. & Buchanan, R. W. (2002) Commentary on the Soteria project: Misguided therapeutics. *Schizophrenia Bulletin*, 28(4), pp.577–581.

Cecil, C. A. M., Viding, E., Fearon, P., Glaser, D. & McCrory, E. J. (2017) Disentangling the mental health impact of childhood abuse and neglect. *Child Abuse & Neglect.* 63, pp.106–119.

Centre For Mental Health (2016) *Missed opportunities: A review of recent evidence into children and young people's mental health.* Available from: https://www.centreformentalhealth.org.uk/missed-opportunities [Accessed 10 March 2017].

Corstens, D., McCarthy-Jones, S., Longden, E. & Thomas, N. (2014) Emerging perspectives from the Hearing Voices Movement: Implications for research and practice. *Schizophrenia Bulletin*, 40(suppl. no. 4), S285–S294.

DOH (2016) *Future in mind: 1 year on.* Available from: https://www.gov.uk/government/speeches/future-in-mind-1-year-on. [Accessed 10 March 2017].

DOH (2015) Future in mind: Promoting, protecting and improving our children and young people's mental health and wellbeing. Available from: https://www.gov.uk/government/uploads/system/uploads/attachment_data/file/414024/Childrens_Mental_Health.pdf [Accessed 10 May 2017].

DOH (2011) *No health without mental health: A cross-governmental outcomes strategy for people of all ages.* London: HMSO. Available from: https://www.gov.uk/government/publications/the-mental-health-strategy-for-england [Accessed 14 November 2017].

DOH (2009) *Department of Health: New Horizons: Towards a shared vision for mental health. Consultation.* London: Department of Health.

EIF (2016) *The cost of late interventions: EIF analysis 2016.* Available from: www.eif.org.uk/publication/the-cost-of-late-intervention-eif-analysis-2016/ [Accessed 10 March 2017].

Fava, G. A. et al. (2001) Long-term outcome of panic disorder with agoraphobia treated by exposure. *Psychological Medicine.* 31(5), pp.891–898.

Goodyer, I. M. et al. (2013) Cognitive behavioural therapy and short-term psychoanalytical psychotherapy versus a brief psychosocial intervention in adolescents with unipolar major depressive disorder (IMPACT): A multicentre, pragmatic, observer-blind, randomised controlled superiority trial. *Lancet Psychiatry* (published online 30 November 2013).

Gottstein, J. (2015) Lessons from Soteria-Alaska. *Mad in America.* Available from: https://www.madinamerica.com/2015/06/lessons-from-soteria-alaska/ [Accessed 10 March 2017].

Greenfield, E. A. & Marks, N. F. (2010) Identifying experiences of physical and psychological violence in childhood that jeopardize mental health in adulthood. *Child Abuse and Neglect*, 34(3), pp.161–171.

Hallam, R. (2015a) *The therapy relationship: A special kind of friendship.* London, Karnac Books.

Hallam, R. (2015b) How should we define practice, client, and professional conduct? *Clinical Psychology Forum*. 270, pp.19–22.

Hallam, R. S. (2013) *Individual case formulation*. Oxford, Academic Press.

Hallam, R. S. and Bender, M. (2011) *David's box: The journals and letters of a young man diagnosed as schizophrenic, 1960–1971*. London, Polpresa Press.

Halmos, P. (1970) *The personal service society*. London, Constable.

Hawton, K., Casañas, I., Comabella, C., Haw, C. & Saunders, K. (2013) Risk factors for suicide in individuals with depression: A systematic review. *Journal of Affective Disorders*, 147, pp.17–28.

HMG (2017) *The Government's response to the Five Year Forward View for Mental Health*. Available from: https://www.gov.uk/government/publications/five-year-forward-view-for-mental-health-government-response [Accessed 10 May 2017].

Hofmann, S. G. & Spiegel, D. A. (1999) Panic control treatment and its applications. *Journal of Psychotherapy Practice and Research*, 8(1), pp.3–11.

Holmes, G. (2010) *Psychology in the real world: Community-based groupwork*. Ross-on-Wye: PCCS Books.

Howard League for Penal Reform (n.d.) 2016 becomes worst year ever recorded for suicides in prisons. Available from: http://howardleague.org/news/suicidesinprison2016/ [Accessed 13 April 2017].

IAPT (2016) *IAPT Annual report, 2015–16*. Available from: http://content.digital.nhs.uk/catalogue/PUB22110/psych-ther-ann-rep-2015-16.pdf [Accessed 10 May 2017].

Joffe, J. M. & Albee, G. W. (1981) *Prevention through political action and social change*. Hanover, NH, University Press of New England.

Johnsen, T. J., & Friborg, O. (2015) The effects of cognitive behavioral therapy as an anti-depressive treatment is falling: A meta-analysis. *Psychological Bulletin*. 141(4), pp.747–768.

Leudar, I. & Thomas, P. (2000) *Voices of reason, voices of insanity*. London, Routledge.

Lomas, T. (2015) Positive social psychology: A multilevel inquiry into sociocultural well-being initiatives. *Psychology Public Policy and Law*, 21(3), pp.338–347.

Longden, E., Corstens, D. & Dillon, J. (2013) Recovery, discovery and revolution: The work of Intervoice and the Hearing Voices Movement. In: Coles, S., Keenan, S. & Diamond, B. (eds.) *Madness contested: Power and practice*, Ross-on-Wye, PCCS Books.

Main, T. (1946) The hospital as a therapeutic institution. *Bulletin of the Menninger Clinic*. 10, pp.66–70.

Maisel, E. (2016) *The future of mental health: Deconstructing the mental disorder paradigm*. New Brunswick, NJ, Transaction.

Maniglio, R. (2012) Child sexual abuse in the etiology of anxiety disorders: A systematic review of reviews. *Trauma, Violence, and Abuse*, 14(2), pp.96–112.

Maniglio, R. (2010) Child sexual abuse in the etiology of depression: A systematic review of reviews. *Depression and Anxiety*, 27(7), pp.631–642.

Marks, I.M., Hallam, R.S., Philpott, R. & Connolly, J. (1976) *Behavioural psychotherapy for nurses: An advanced clinical role for nurses*. London, RCN Research Series.

McCarthy-Jones, S. (2017) *Can't you hear them? The science and significance of hearing voices*. London, Jessica Kingsley.

McElroy, S., & Hevey, D. (2014) Relationship between adverse early experiences, stressors, psychosocial resources and wellbeing. *Child Abuse & Neglect*. 38(1), pp.65–75.

McKnight, J. (1995) *The careless society: Community and its counterfeits*. New York, Basic Books.

Mersky, J. P., Topitzes, J. & Reynolds, A. J. (2013) Impacts of adverse childhood experiences on health, mental health, and substance use in early adulthood: A cohort study of an urban, minority sample in the U.S. *Child Abuse and Neglect*. 37(11), pp.917–925.

Miret. M., Ayuso-Mateos, J. L., Sanchez-Moreno. J. & Vieta, E. (2013) Depressive disorders and suicide: Epidemiology, risk factors, and burden. *Neuroscience and Biobehavioral Reviews*. 37, pp.2372–2374.

Mosher, L. & Burti, L. (1994) *Community mental health*. New York: W. W. Norton.

Mosher, L. R., Hendrix, V. & Fort, D. C. (2004) *Soteria: Through madness to deliverance*. Bloomington, IN, Xlibris.

New Savoy Partnership (n.d) NSP/BPS Staff wellbeing charter. Available from: www.newsavoypartnership.org/nsp-bps-staff-wellbeing-charter.htm [Accessed 10 March 2017].

NHS (2016) *Five year forward view for mental health: A report from the independent Mental Health Taskforce to the NHS in England*. Available from: https://www.england.nhs.uk/wp-content/uploads/2016/02/Mental-Health-Taskforce-FYFV-final.pdf [Accessed 10 March 2017].

ONS (2014) *Suicides in the United Kingdom*. London, Office for National Statistics, Statistical Bulletin. Available from: www.ons.gov.uk [Accessed 10 November 2016].

Osburn, J. (2006) An overview of social role valorization theory. *The SRV Journal*. 1(1), pp.4–13.

Pearson, D. & Baboulene, K. (2016) Soteria Brighton: Origins and activities. *Asylum*. 23(2), pp.18–19.

PHE (Public Health England) (2017) Psychosocial pathways and health outcomes: Informing action on health inequalities. Available from: https://www.gov.uk/government/uploads/system/uploads/attachment_data/file/640674/20170824_Psychosocial_pathways_and_health_equity.pdf [Accessed 10 September 2017].

Pollak, S. (2016) Adversities in childhood and their impact on mental health across the life course. *European Psychiatry*. 33, S1.

Proctor, G. (2015) The NHS in 2015: Still a scary possibility to come. *Healthcare Counselling & Psychotherapy Journal*. October, pp.9–14. Available from: www.bacp.co.uk/docs/pdf/14632_feature%20article%20hcpj%20oct%2015.pdf [Accessed 10 May 2017].

Pugh, N. E., Hadjistavropoulos, H. D., Klein, B. & Austin, D. W. (2014) A case study illustrating therapist assisted internet cognitive behavior therapy for depression. *Cognitive and Behavioral Practice*, 21, pp.64–77.

Rao, A. S., Bhutani, G., Dosanjh, N., Clarke, J., Hacker-Hughes, J., Easton, E., Van Laar, D., Cohen-Tovée, E. (2016) *Psychological wellbeing and resilience: Resetting the balance*. Available from: www.bps.org.uk/system/files/Public%20files/ar_v10_resetting_the_balance_160516.docx.pdf [Accessed 10 May 2017].

Read, J., Fosse, R., Moskowitz, A. & Perry, B. (2014) The traumagenic neurodevelopmental model of psychosis revisited. *Neuropsychiatry*. 4(1), pp.65–79.

Rogers, A. & Pilgrim, D. (1993) Service users' views of psychiatric treatments. *Sociology of Health & Illness*. 15(5), pp.612–631.

Romme, M. & Escher, S. (2009) *Living with voices: 50 voices of recovery*. Ross-on-Wye: PCCS Books.

Saxena, S. & Setoya, Y. (2014) World Health Organization's comprehensive mental health action plan 2013–2020. *Psychiatry and Clinical Neurosciences*. 68, pp.585–586.

Seikkula, J. (2011) Becoming dialogical: Psychotherapy or a way of life? *The Australian and New Zealand Journal of Family Therapy*. 32(3), pp.179–193.

Seikkula, J. (2006) Five-year experience of first-episode non-affective psychosis in open-dialogue approach. *Psychotherapy Research*. 16, pp.214–228.

Seikkula, J., Alakare, B., & Aaltonen, J. (2011) The comprehensive open-dialogue approach (II): Long-term stability of acute psychosis outcomes in advanced community care: The Western Lapland project. *Psychosis*. 3, pp.192–204.

Sharman, J. (2017) Using children's mental health funding to plug NHS gaps is 'like theft', says former health minister. *Independent*, 9 January. www.independent.co.uk/news/uk/politics/nhs-funding-children-mental-health-cash-jeremy-hunt-theft-norman-lamb-lib-dem-theresa-may-a7516806.html [Accessed 28 November 2017].

Shaw, B. (2013) Peer support. In: Coles, S., Keenan, S. & Diamond, B. (eds.) *Madness contested: Power and practice*. Ross-on-Wye: PCCS Books, pp.293–306.

Silcox, S. (2009) Nearly one in 10 European workers report work-related health problems. *Occupational Health*. 61(10), p.31.

Soteria Network UK. Available from: www.soterianetwork.org.uk/local/index.html [Accessed 10 November 2016].

Stafford, M., Catharine R. Gale, C. R., Mishra, G., Richards., Black, S. & Kuh, D. L. (2015) Childhood environment and mental wellbeing at age 60–64 years: Prospective evidence from the MRC National Survey of Health and Development. *PLoS ONE*, 10(6), e0126683. doi:10.1371/journal.pone.0126683.

Susskind, R. & Susskind, D. (2015) *The future of the professions: How technology will transform the work of human experts*. Oxford, Oxford University Press.

Szasz, T. (1981) On preventing psychopathology: A libertarian analysis. In: Joffe, J. M. & Albee, G. W. (1981) *Prevention through political action and social change*. Hanover, NH, University Press of New England, pp.26–33.

Thoits, P. A. (2016) 'I'm not mentally ill'. Identity deflection as a form of stigma and resistance. *Journal of Health and Social Behavior*. 57(2), pp.135–151.

Thoits, P. A. (2010) Stress and health: Major findings and policy implications. *Journal of Health and Social Behavior*. 51, Suppl. S41–53.

Walker, P. (2017) More than 350 Sure Start centres have closed since 2010. *The Guardian*, 2 February. Available from: https://www.theguardian.com/society/2017/feb/02/sure-start-centres-300-closed-since-2010 [Accessed 28 November 2017].

White, J. (2008) Stepping up primary care. *The Psychologist*, 21(10), pp.844–847.

WHO (2017) Suicide Fact sheet. Available from: www.who.int/mediacentre/factsheets/fs398/en/ [Accessed 14 November 2016].

WHO (2013) World Health Organization comprehensive mental health action plan 2013–2020. Geneva: WHO. Available from: www.who.int/mental_health/action_plan_2013/en/ [Accessed 10 November 2016].

INDEX

www.ingramcontent.com/pod-product-compliance
Ingram Content Group UK Ltd.
Pitfield, Milton Keynes, MK11 3LW, UK
UKHW011016180926
475701UK00004B/771
* 9 7 8 1 1 3 8 0 6 3 1 3 6 *